84049

D1168658

Learning Resources Center
Collin County Community College District
SPRING CREEK CAMPUS
Plano, Texas 75074

WITHDRAWN

SCC LIBRARY

RA   Devereux, Godfrey.
781.7
D478   15-minute yoga.
2000

$14.95

BAKER & TAYLOR

15-Minute Yoga

15-Minute Yoga

Godfrey Devereux

Thorsons

Thorsons

An Imprint of HarperCollins*Publishers*

77–85 Fulham Palace Road,

Hammersmith, London W6 8JB

The Thorsons website address is:

www.thorsons.com

First published 2000

10 9 8 7 6 5 4 3 2 1

© Godfrey Devereux, 2000

Godfrey Devereux asserts his moral right to

be identified as the author of this work

Cover photographs © Sarah Robbie

A catalogue record for this book

is available from the British Library

ISBN 0 7225 3966 5

Printed and bound in Great Britain by

Woolnough Bookbinding Ltd, Irthlingborough, Northamptonshire

All rights reserved. No part of this publication may be

reproduced, stored in a retrieval system, or transmitted,

in any form or by any means, electronic, mechanical,

photocopying, recording or otherwise, without the prior

permission of the publishers.

Contents

This book is dedicated to the memory of

Derek Ireland

whose honest, grounded presence
immediately dissolved the nonsense and
mystique that surround, and obscure, the simple
practice of yoga, and whose inspiration as
teacher, guide, and friend led so many to a
deeper and richer life.

Acknowledgments

I would like to acknowledge the students and teachers of the Life Centre 1993–1996 for contributing so much to my understanding of the method of hatha yoga.

I would also like to acknowledge the generosity, understanding, patience, and tolerance of Louise White for giving me that possibility.

I would like to thank Belinda Budge for establishing and sustaining a productive relationship with me as my editor.

Preface

It is no surprise that yoga has lasted thousands of years. Nor is it any surprise that its popularity is surging. Pop stars, waiters, actors, secretaries, lawyers, doctors, car mechanics, housewives, athletes—yoga appeals to everyone. It is no longer a cranky pursuit. Instead it is fast becoming the most sought after of exercise and training programs. The reason is simple. Yoga reaches parts that other forms of exercise cannot even contemplate. It exercises every muscle in the body; it tones and invigorates every organ; it flushes and cleans every blood vessel; it pacifies, tones, and harmonizes the nerves; it massages the brain; it realigns bones; it improves posture; it irrigates all body tissues; it enhances skin quality; it clears and relaxes the mind; it focuses attention; it generates energy.

The practice has lasted so long, and is in such demand, simply because it is brilliant—brilliant for the body, brilliant for the mind, a brilliant way to enhance your life. There is no other form of exercise, or any other kind of training, that is so comprehensive. While its method is mainly physical, its effects are not. It enhances the activity of the mind just as much as it does that of the body. It does so with the utmost simplicity. It requires no special machinery or gadgets; it needs no specialist understanding. All you need to practice yoga is a body, a mind, a little floor space, a little bit of time, and motivation. We can all have that. Once you start to practice its benefits are so immediately obvious that it becomes easier and easier to find both the time and the motivation to continue. There is no need to impose a strenuous discipline on yourself. It's just a matter of going to your mat and doing it.

Doing yoga could hardly be more simple. In fact it is a very natural process, especially first thing in the morning: cats do it, dogs do it, children do it. In fact most of us, even now, still do it. We wake up, and we stretch: an arm or two, a leg or two. On the surface yoga is simply organized stretching—a stretching of the whole body undertaken systematically, regularly, and consistently. The remarkable power of yoga comes from the way we go about the stretch (the internal dynamic), and the organization of the different stretches into sequences (the external dynamic) that open, relax, and tone the body gently, gradually, safely, and effectively.

The internal dynamic and the external dynamic are equally important. Together they transform yoga from a flexibility training into a whole body/whole mind training that has the power to enhance your life enormously. It is much more than simply developing fitness while becoming more relaxed, although yoga does both of these more effectively than any other training. You can become flexible, relaxed, stronger, more alert, fitter, focused, and full of vitality—all with a little diligent cross-training. But yoga has a magic ingredient that is unique. Most importantly of all yoga will help you become more comfortable with yourself. As you become more comfortable in your body, and more at ease in your mind, you will feel better and better about yourself. This is the secret of yoga. It is not about becoming a better person by becoming a different person. It is about becoming better about being the person that you are. It helps you to drop the tensions, anxieties, and inhibitions that prevent you from being fully and freely yourself. It teaches you to like and love yourself.

You do this in yoga simply by paying attention to the way your body feels as you move it, to the rhythm of your breathing, in and out of different postures. Nothing weird, nothing esoteric, nothing complicated. Just moving, breathing, and feeling. With, again, one secret ingredient—staying still, and breathing and feeling. While how you move in and out of the postures is important, it is the staying still that really counts. It is this that distinguishes yoga from other forms of training: giving yourself time to stop still, to listen to your body, to feel yourself as you are.

You are going to be amazed and delighted by how simple yoga is. And you are going to be amazed and delighted at how much you are going to get out of it.

Introduction

Yoga is a practice of moving with the breath into stillness. The stillness takes place within specific shapes: the yoga postures. These postures are varied in their shapes and their familiarity. Many of them can be seen in the everyday activity of children, athletes, dancers, and gymnasts. Some of them cannot. The more advanced yoga postures can be very extreme in the demands that they put upon muscles, joints, and ligaments. However the benefits of yoga are not in proportion to the difficulty of the postures. Most of the benefits of yoga result from the more basic postures. The advanced postures simply add a little delicious icing to the basic nutrition of the cake.

The benefits do not come simply from making the body take a specific shape. Yoga is not like dance or gymnastics. Even though many yoga postures are very beautiful, the way that a posture looks is not the point. Yoga is not an external practice. It is an *internal* one. The point is the inner dynamic that sustains the posture in an effortless stillness. This is dynamic stillness, or meditative action. It requires the presence of the mind. Paying attention to the breath brings the mind into the equation and changes the shapes of the postures into powerful tools of transformation.

The mind is brought to bear on the inner activity that sustains the outer shape of the posture. Without presence of mind the inner activity will be incomplete and then so too will be the posture. Then it will not be able to provide all of its benefits. The basic yoga postures require a contribution from each part of the body. It is not just a question of moving the spine. The spine must be supported by the pelvis, legs, and feet. It must be assisted by the chest, neck, arms, and hands. The shapes become yoga postures by involving all of the body and all of the mind.

One of the drawbacks of words is that they create divisions. The spine is the spine, not the legs. The legs are the legs but not the arms. Of course this is true. However the body does not work within itself in the same way that words do. Although it is clear from the outside that arms are arms and legs legs, from within it is not so clear. When we raise an arm the muscles in the legs and feet are also changed in their activity. If it were not so we would lose our balance. So, as far as the body is concerned, the absolute distinction that words make between body parts and muscles does not hold. This becomes very clear in yoga. When the spine is under stress and needs relief, we often have to change the activity of the legs while doing nothing directly with the spine. Likewise the line and position of the pelvis is secured by adjusting the feet and the legs. In yoga the body is a whole. The parts are not separable. The activity of each part determines and is determined by the activity of every other part. The mind, too, is a vital part of this equation. It is needed to re-educate muscular relationships that have become dormant or restricted through years of bad habit.

This fact underlies the way that the postures must be approached. Just as the body has its innate integrity that goes deeper than the separation of various parts, so too does the method of the practice. While the shapes of the postures can easily be approximated without the integrity of this approach, their benefits will be compromised. To access the full range and depth of its benefits the practice of yoga must be approached with integrity. This integrity is one in which the attentiveness and sensitivity of the mind are used to activate and integrate each part of the body into a harmonious whole. This is a harmony of both body and mind: as one. The guiding link is the breath.

What this means is that yoga is not simply a matter of establishing the greatest possible movement in a muscle or muscle group. Yoga is not a fancy form of stretching. It is not simply a matter of lengthening muscles: it is a question of retuning all the muscles of the body and their relationships to each other. This retuning is not done in order to bring about flexibility. It is done in order to bring about efficiency and harmony of all physical activity. This is not just about muscular movement. It is also a question of the organic activity of the vital systems of the body: respiratory, circulatory, digestive, reproductive, immunological, nervous, etc. Nevertheless, flexibility is an obvious and beneficial effect of this process. But it is important to realize that flexibility is not the be all and end all of yoga: nor are strength, stamina or any combination thereof. Yoga is *not* primarily fitness training, though it will make you fit.

The more you put into the practice of yoga the more you will get out of it. It can be used to develop flexibility, strength, stamina, and general fitness. It can be used to promote relaxation and good posture. It can be used to correct muscular imbalances and skeletal defects. It can be used to overcome illness and prevent disease. But it can give much more than these things, while including them also. It can give a deep and resilient peace of mind, which comes from self-awareness and self-acceptance that rest upon the self-determination and self-responsibility which the method demands. No-one can do your practice for you. Once you begin to feel the way that it opens you to yourself, allowing you to feel and be yourself more fully and more freely, you will greatly appreciate this fact.

Introduction

Caution

Yoga asks your muscles to works in new and unfamiliar ways. These ways are neither unnatural nor harmful. However they must be approached with caution, especially if you have any current or old injuries, or if you are ill, recovering from illness, pregnant, exhausted or actively compromised in any other way. This book outlines the way to approach the practice of the yoga postures so that they are safe, accessible, and effective. It is important that the guidelines given are followed exactly as outlined. Failure to do so may result in strain or injury.

Yoga is not just a technical process. It also has an inner dimension. This inner dimension is in fact far more important to your overall well-being than the mechanical techniques of the postures. While the correct technique protects your body from injury, it cannot protect your mind. The effect that yoga has on your mind, and therefore on your everyday life (and in particular your relationships), depends much more on your motivation and your attitude.

The effect that practice has on your state of mind depends almost entirely on these two factors in combination. The wrong motivation and attitude can create an aggression in the mind that is harnessed and amplified through the practice. It is not so much that wanting to become superflexible, superman strong, or supermodel skinny is harmful. It is what that motivation can do to the attitude that you bring to the practice. It can make you push yourself beyond your safe limits. It can encourage you to force muscles, to strain joints, to damage ligaments. More seriously your ambition to achieve a preconceived result can constantly give you a sense of your own inadequacy as you are. Then while your practice may make you more flexible and stronger, and you might feel good about that, on a deeper level you are undermining your self-esteem, and your self-confidence.

To avoid this deadly pitfall you require two constant allies: sensitivity and honesty. You must apply sensitivity to what you are doing so that you can be honestly aware of the effect it is having on you, and not only on your body but also on your mind. Is what you are doing making you feel more relaxed about yourself, or is it making you aggressive, impatient, or irritable? We all have our limits: so too does each part of us; every muscle, every ligament, every joint. We must respect these limits, moment by moment. This does not mean we consign ourselves to their limitations forever. Not at all. It means that we should explore and express those limits with sensitivity and honesty, so that they can expand, so that you can grow according to your current capacity. With this motivation and attitude the application of the correct technique to the practice of yoga postures will result not only in enjoyable physical benefits, but deeply satisfying psychological benefits too. Yoga practiced with an honest sensitivity to your limitations, and their innate impulse to expand, will result in a deepening of your self-esteem and nourishing of your self-confidence that far outweighs the more obvious physical benefits.

Caution

How to Use this Book

This book has been written and designed to make it possible for anyone with normal mobility to learn yoga safely, easily, and effectively. It is divided into four sections: **Theory, Method, Practice,** and **Postures**. Theory without practice is useless, while practice without theory is dangerous. Therefore, please read the theoretical section *first*. In it you will find the guidance that you need to create for yourself a safe and effective context within which to practice. This consists of an understanding of the method of the practice: what it does, how it does it and what it leads to. The **Practice** section should be read thoroughly before starting to practice. It includes a brief **Anatomy of Yoga** to help you with the postures.

The method of hatha yoga is very specific. In essence it is very simple, but in practice can be a little daunting. Every effort has been made to capture and clarify its simplicity in the theoretical section. However, if you want to go a little deeper into the underlying principles and their application, you will benefit from reading the technical section of my *Dynamic Yoga*, published by Thorsons. This gives a detailed presentation of the technicalities of the hatha yoga method.

The **Posture** section of the book is divided into six sections. Each section consists of a group of postures, followed by a practice sequence. Each section is named after the effect of the postures outlined there. The postures are numbered within each section, and each one also has a letter that refers to the section in which it is defined and detailed. For example postures detailed in the first section are energizing postures and have designated **E** numbers, such as **E1**, **E2**, etc. Not all of the postures in a practice sequence are detailed in that particular section. You will have to refer to other sections to locate them.

You may use the individual sections in the practical part of the book in any order that you like, according to your need. You may feel a need to begin with the **Energizing Practice** and stay with that only for a while, before proceeding to another practice. Or you may prefer to try them all out, one after another so that you can choose which one to practice on the basis of your direct experience of them.

All of the practice sequences can be done in 15 minutes. They can also take longer if you go more slowly, and hold some or all of the postures for longer times, or repeat them. With the exception of the **Balancing Practice**, one minute is the average time given to a posture, or to one side of a posture that is done on each side. This is an arbitrary figure. You can change the effect of a posture practice by changing the speed at which you work. Working faster will charge you up more. Working slower will chill you out more. But, when you want to energize more and go faster, *do not hurry*. Always proceed at a pace that allows you to approach the postures with care and sensitivity. The only safeguard you have against strain or injury is your own attentiveness. The **Balancing Practice** is longer than the others, with less time given to complete each posture if it is done in 15 minutes. Wait until you have tried all the other sequences, and are familiar with all the postures, before attempting it in that time.

How to Use this Book

When undertaking the practice of a particular sequence, first read through the instructions for all of the postures to give yourself an overview of where you will be going. Then, using the two-page spread of the sequence as a guide, go through the practice posture by posture, referring back to the detailed instructions for each posture as closely and faithfully as you can. The first few times that you try a sequence allow a little more time than 15 minutes to help you find your way without rushing.

Always give a little time to lying down at the end of your practice to allow mind and body to assimilate its effects. When you are familiar with the sequences and find you have more time available you can combine the different sequences. To do this effectively you will have to modify them somewhat so that you are following a balanced and safe practice sequence.

When your love of yoga requires longer and more challenging practices you will benefit from *Dynamic Yoga* (G. Devereux, published by Thorsons).

PART ONE

Theory

The theory of yoga must be understood if its practice is to be fruitful. Even though yoga is in fact very simple, and quite natural, it is unfamiliar. This unfamiliarity can make it difficult to correctly apply the techniques. Especially because the way that we use our bodies is always to some extent unbalanced and, therefore restrictive. Also because the way we use our bodies is such a deeply ingrained part of our sense of who we are. This makes it quite difficult to change the way we use our bodies. This is not because yoga is unnatural or difficult; it is simply because the power of physical and psychological habit that underlies our use of the body is so great. Little by little yoga undermines that power, releases the body from its distortions, and gives access to the far greater power of the body's intrinsic integrity. In order for this to occur it is important to understand what is behind the techniques: the theory of yoga.

2

WHAT YOGA IS

Yoga is a training method, not a religion. You are not required to have any special beliefs, ideals or aspirations in order to practice or benefit from yoga. If anything it is more like science than religion. It is a way of finding things out. In yoga you discover the possibilities of your true potential. This occurs both on a physical and a non-physical level. Physically it is a method of developing the potential of the human body to its highest level. This goes far beyond simply developing fitness. It also develops organic health through its effect on the internal organs. At the same time, by developing the sensitivity of the nervous system, it also enhances sensory potential. This means that sight, hearing, taste, smell, and touch become more acute. This is not only more rewarding but also brings us into more direct, accurate, and intimate contact with the world and our life. At a certain level this enhanced sensory perception can appear almost magical. It can give the impression that the unseen can be seen, the inaudible can be heard. Whereas, in fact, it is more a question of lowering the threshold of perception so that what is normally missed or filtered out is received and retained.

Yoga is also more like technology than religion as it is a way of making things happen. It does not simply reveal the possibilities of our potential — it actually activates the potential lying within us, enhancing the range of possibilities open to us. Yoga empowers us to live a deeper, richer, more satisfying life, simply by awakening what is already within us. This process is not dependent on any special skill, training or talent. It does not require specialist esoteric or scientific knowledge. We do not have to know anything about our dormant potential. The practice of yoga itself is the means for accessing what is already there. It is simply a question of removing the veils, opening the door.

The veils are removed by the simple process of relaxing. The yoga training method is designed to bring about total relaxation. It is only the presence of physical, emotional, and mental tension that restricts the flowering of our innate potential. As these tensions are removed, our potential is realized accordingly. Yoga is designed to strip away these tensions, one by one: slowly, safely, and permanently. When they are all gone, and we are totally relaxed, our full potential is free to express itself unhindered. As the natural harmony and integrity of our body and mind are more able to express themselves, the more immune we become to the stress and strain of life. While we cannot avoid the difficulties and problems that life contains, we can and do learn to navigate them safely, in order to live free from tension and anxiety.

Yoga enables us to do this as a matter of course. We do not have to develop a special strategy for coping with life. We do not need to be prepared for everything before it happens. The practice of yoga stabilizes our nervous system and our minds. This stability spills over into our lives allowing us to face the unexpected with a calm clarity. This is the essence of the meditative mind.

Yoga is not separate from meditation. In fact meditation is simply one aspect of yoga. It is the core and the fruit of yoga. Meditation has two aspects: the method and the effect, the process and the result. The practices of yoga are the meditative method, the meditative process. They require and cultivate deep and acute presence of mind. Living in the equanimity of a stable mind is the effect, the result of yoga. It is something that can be enjoyed as a result of the practice, both within the practice itself and in every aspect of normal, daily life.

It is only a very specialist kind of meditation that requires withdrawal from life. This is a meditation that uses intense concentration and which requires

4

total freedom from distraction. More useful to the living of a normal, daily life is meditation that uses awareness. This kind of meditation does not need an absence of stimulus. It uses the stimulus of physical and mental activity as a tool to develop a meditative state. This kind of meditation, which is at the heart of the yoga method, is one in which awareness of that which is occurring is clarified, intensified, deepened, and stabilized to the extent that it becomes the ongoing state of mind. It is not a special state which requires silence and special rituals to enter. It is an ongoing state of being in which all activities are not only possible but greatly enhanced.

Yoga practice then is dynamic meditation. To practice yoga effectively is to practice meditation. This is not hindered even by the most intensely physical aspects of yoga. Quite the reverse. The physicality of the method challenges our awareness to maintain stability and clarity under practical duress. It empowers us to retain a meditative state even in the midst of intense pressure. In fact the process of progression through the yoga practices, both the postures and the breathing techniques, can be better understood from this perspective. It is not a matter of needing or trying to develop super flexibility, or the ability to hold the breath for minutes at a time. The advanced postures and breathing practices are designed primarily as challenges to the mind, not as means to develop magical physical capabilities. They cultivate and refine the ability of the mind to remain calm, stable, and lucid under extremes of stress. For make no mistake about it, the advanced yoga techniques are difficult. To a body and mind unprepared they will be a source of stress. To ones well-prepared through the preliminary practices, and sufficiently stabilized as a result, they become a potent means to enhance that stability—to access more fully and more easily a meditative state of mind.

It is the ability to cultivate the meditative mind, and to live from it, that releases our non-physical potential. This includes improving the activity of

5

the mind: memory, perception, understanding, reason, intuition. It also includes our emotional well-being. We become more tranquil, more balanced, less anxious, less needy. It also has an impact on our spiritual nature. It allows the richness of our spirituality to emerge. It gives us a deep sense of connectedness and belonging, which bring with them compassion, peace of mind, and joy. This is, again, not a question of having to follow some special scheme of being or action. It is a quite natural result of authentic practice. For yoga is, at heart, a spiritual practice. Its impact on body and mind, remarkable as it is, is simply a side effect. The basic purpose is to free us from the ignorance and restrictions that limit the full and free expression of our spiritual nature. It is this effect that causes the mistaken association of yoga with religion. Whereas in fact yoga allows individuals to actually achieve on their own what religions promise but rarely deliver.

HOW YOGA WORKS

Yoga works in a very simple but very effective way. By moving the body in and out of a variety of different postures, and holding still in them, the body is recalibrated. This process involves the whole of the body, and the mind as well. It is not just a question of stretching muscles to become more flexible. The muscles are utilized in very definite and deliberate ways that rearrange and restructure the whole body, including the vital organs.

There are hundreds of muscles in the human body. Many of them do not even have names. We are aware of only a very few of them. Each muscle can function within a number of different muscle groups to bring about a particular action. A muscle then is a little bit like a letter in the alphabet. It has its own character and location, but it can act in many different ways, depending on which other muscles it is cooperating with.

Yoga is designed not just to reach every individual muscle. It also sets out to recalibrate all the different muscular relationships that are possible to the human body. Most of these possibilities are never even used in our lives. We move and live in such a limited way compared to our innate capability. Yoga seeks to access and release that capability as much as possible. Then we become free to live a richer, more satisfying life.

Yoga goes about this by putting the body into postures that are designed to open the joints of the body at the same time as lengthening the muscles. This makes it very different from stretch exercise, which is concerned only with muscle length. The muscles are used to establish the bones in positions in which the joints can be opened. There are of course many joints in the body. Every vertebra in the spine is a joint. Then there are the more obvious ones: wrists, elbows, shoulders, ankles, knees, hips. But there are many more: where the pubic bones join; where they join to the pelvis;

7

where the sacrum attaches to the pelvis; the joints in fingers and toes. Luckily it is not necessary to know all of the joints and their location in order to open them. The postures take care of that—provided they are done in the correct way.

While stretching is an obvious part of yoga it is a means not an end. Many muscles cause restriction or imbalance in a joint because of tightness, or because of weakness. Those muscles that are tight need to be loosened, i.e. stretched, while those muscles that are weak need to be strengthened, i.e. toned. So yoga is also about toning and strengthening muscles. This strengthening is a very different kind to the strengthening developed in weight training. It is not based on increasing bulk. It is based on increasing efficiency. Rather than increasing the number of muscle fibers it increases the capacity of those that already exist. So muscles do not get much bigger, they simply become more toned. Rather than using repetitive pumping actions to increase bulk, yoga utilizes sustained supporting actions to increase efficiency. This makes it much less demanding, much less tiring than other forms of exercise. In fact yoga is deeply rejuvenating and re-energizing.

The sustained supporting activity utilized in yoga is not just designed to develop muscular efficiency. It is designed to create and maintain space in the joints: to help the joints to open. By developing the capacity to hold the body still in specific postures, the muscles are able to allow the tendons, ligaments, and bones of the body to establish new relationships with each other. The yoga postures are designed to ensure that these new relationships are the optimum ones for both the structural and functional aspects of the body.

On the surface this means that each muscle is brought to a peak of tone and flexibility. For this to happen the yoga postures have to work deeply into every muscle of the body, and into every relationship that can exist between all the individual muscles. They have to rid the body completely of muscular tension. This they can do, although to completely free the body from tension would mean using the hundreds of yoga postures that exist, not just the 30-odd explained here! However most of the work is done by a basic group of about 60 postures. The remaining postures simply refine and maintain the work of the core postures.

Our bodies are full of tension. That tension has been with us from day one. It is a part of who we think we are. It is a deeply ingrained part of our sense of our self, which is very much determined by our physical capability and tendencies. It is no easy thing then to release the body from tension. It requires commitment, perseverance and patience. Most of the tension that we carry is the result of some kind of past shock to the body or mind. It is the leftover of a difficult moment or situation that is still unresolved. The tension is the expression of that lack of resolution. Yoga sets out to bring about the complete resolution of unresolved tension, by working on physical, mental, *and* emotional release. There will be some unresolved feeling related to the majority of areas of physical tension in the body. Releasing the physical tension releases the unresolved feeling. This can be a very satisfying process: it brings with it a deep sense of release and relief. This is often accompanied by an urge to cry. Some people find this strange and shocking and resist it. This should not be done. The tears are tears of relief, they are nothing to be ashamed or afraid of. They should be welcomed as a sign of progress.

Besides bringing about physical freedom and emotional release, yoga also causes energetic amplification. This means that it tends to enhance whatever state you bring to it. If you bring aggression to your practice it makes you even more aggressive. If you bring openness, it enhances your openness. If you bring sensitivity it enhances your sensitivity. This is a very important point to bear in mind. Yoga is not a competitive sport. It is far more sophisticated and subtle than any other form of human activity. It is very powerful. It will have a strong effect on anyone. It is important to make sure that the effect it brings is beneficial. Treat it as a gift to yourself, a luxurious treat that is going to bring you closer to yourself, and allow you to live a richer, more fulfilling life. Do not approach it as if it were some kind of spartan discipline, some ascetic self-mortification. This will just turn your practice into a whipping stick that will drive you deeper and deeper into aggression, denial, and frustration.

Yoga also works on the mind. Our mind is to a great extent conditioned by the information we have been receiving through our senses since before birth. This information is brought to the brain by the nerves to be processed. The nerves that bring this information are the sensory/motor nerves. They are not the sensory nerves. They are the sensory *and* motor nerves. The nerves that carry commands to the muscles also carry feedback from the world. This is at the very heart of yoga's power. By developing, recalibrating, and refining the muscles through the nervous system, the sensory pathways of the nervous system are also being developed, recalibrated, and refined. Just by moving in and out of postures, and holding them. The body and mind are not just two separate things. They are also a single continuum. What happens to the body happens also to the mind.

A quick glance at child development shows that human intelligence is dependent on movement. The child uses movement to bring it into contact with the world as fully and deeply as possible. This movement brings about sensory development, which in turn brings about development of intelligence. The yoga postures clarify, develop, and increase the connections between the motor nerves throughout the brain. Because the nerves feeding these brain cells are also sensory nerves, the postures also clarify, develop, and refine the sensory centers of the brain. This allows for a much richer, clearer, and more accurate awareness of the world. Yoga makes you more perceptive, more aware, more awake to life.

11

Theory

WHAT YOGA DOES

The effects of yoga are very broad and very deep. They touch every aspect of one's being, every aspect of one's life. Most immediately they give back the capability of the body to move freely and effortlessly. At the same time they give the mind focus, while bringing a vitality and enthusiasm for life that is priceless.

The precise alignment of the body required by the postures brings, little by little, structural reintegration to the anatomical body. Posture, the way that we hold ourselves, improves; carriage, the way that we move through space, does too. The muscles of the body are all more able to fulfill their role in supporting and moving the rest of the body once they are free from tension. The same is true when all of their fibers are functioning at peak capacity. Both result from consistent yoga practice. This means that simple processes—of resisting gravity to stand up, moving the body in simple actions—no longer come at a price. These simple, natural processes are no longer bringing stress, wear, and tear to the body. When all the muscles are functionally efficient and free from tension each one is able to make its contribution to the body's activity without stress or strain.

Simple, everyday activities become easier, effortless. This not only makes the body something that gives pleasure even in the simplest activity. It also means that it gets tired much less easily. The tasks and pleasures of life no longer bring fatigue and exhaustion. We recover our capacity for continuous activity when that activity is no longer stressful. Along with this physical stamina comes the mental equivalent. The ability of the mind to stay focused on simple unexciting activities gives it a perseverance it can bring to any and all activities. The distracting thoughts that undermine our capacity to complete necessary but unstimulating activities are less frequent and have less power. So we are more able to complete these tasks happily and contentedly.

Yoga does not only work on an anatomical level. It works deeply on the physiological activity of the body. The way it does so is as thorough as it is simple. The basis of yoga practice is to breathe freely while moving slowly with awareness. This immediately stimulates respiration and blood circulation. Not only does blood circulate more freely, but it is more fully oxygenated. It brings more fuel to nourish the body cells. This benefit reaches every cell in the body; they are all able to convert nutrients into energy and replacement materials better. The deep stretching that yoga brings to the muscles, and the effect of improved circulation, bring oxygenated blood to tissues that may have been neglected due to poor circulation. Those parts of the body that have been or are beginning to stagnate, are brought back to life, to vitality.

Just as respiration and circulation are improved, so too is digestion. As the cells of the digestive organs are more efficiently replaced and nourished, their activity improves. The movement of food and nutrients through the digestive canal is also enhanced by the anatomical impact of the postures. The postures bring about a deep, slow, and sustained internal massage on the internal organs: compressing, stretching, squeezing this part of the body and then that. This internal massage stimulates the flow of blood deep into the organs, cleansing them of old, stagnant blood, ridding them of waste products, and bringing them oxygen and nutrients. As most of the internal organs are made of muscle tissue their fibers also benefit from the postures just as the larger voluntary muscles do. Yoga works in just the same way to purify and vitalize the reproductive organs.

Enhancement of muscular activity, respiration, circulation, and digestion has a marked psychological and cosmetic effect. Skin color and tone improves. Eyes shine. Posture and bearing improve. This brings about an enhanced sense of well-being, confidence, and self-esteem. All of these things together combine to give the seasoned yoga practitioner a radiance, a glow of vitality, that is more attractive and more valuable than all the offerings of the fashion and cosmetics industries combined.

While improved respiration, circulation, and digestion obviously contribute greatly to improved health, yoga works directly on the immune system too. The various lymph glands, ducts, and organs of the immune system are also subject to improved nutrient and oxygen availability and the effects of deep internal massage. Consequently the ability of the immune system to detect and deal with alien substances is greatly improved. This process is supported by the overall increase in energy and vitality that yoga brings to the body as a whole. Yoga then becomes a generalized and ongoing form of preventative health care. In the right hands it can also be used as a therapy for a large number of illnesses besides obvious structural problems.

Last, but far from least, yoga enhances the activity of the nervous system. Modern life is extremely stressful. Most of us live lives full of pressure. As a result stress (and stress-related illness) is one of the major medical problems of our times. The intricate balance between the various aspects of the nervous system are disturbed by continuous stress. Most of us live in a state known as the "flight/fight mechanism." This means that the active, external, energizing aspect of our nervous system is constantly stimulated and functioning, while the passive, internal, relaxing aspect is neglected. This can lead to a situation in which even when there is no stressor to deal with, even when we have the opportunity to relax, we cannot. Our sympathetic nervous system, which rouses us to effective action, is permanently on, while our parasympathetic nervous system, which calms, relaxes, and reju- venates us, is turned off. Yoga rectifies this imbalance. The way that we move and act during yoga, and the attitude of open, sensitive exploration that we bring to it, stimulate the parasympathetic nervous system, relieving the sympathetic system. We then start to calm down on a very deep level and are able to drop our continual need for action and stimulation.

A major key to this process is the slow, smooth, effortless breathing that yoga encourages.

Yoga utilizes the nervous system completely differently from the way that most activities do. It uses actions and activities that are natural and normal and require no props or special gadgets to reverse the usual activity of the nervous system. Instead of utilizing the stimulating sympathetic nerves, it uses the calming parasympathetic nerves. Moreover, rather than directing the nervous system outwards through the sensory/motor nerves, it turns the sensory/motor nerves and awareness inwards. Eventually this has a powerful impact, both on the nerves and brain, and on the mind. Slowly but surely the mind becomes less hooked on external, vigorous stimuli. Instead it becomes familiar and comfortable with more subtle, internal activity. This makes the mind less intense, less grasping, less neurotic. At the same time the neural activity of the brain is pacified; the brain becomes softer, calmer and more responsive.

By both enhancing the activity of the receptors and pathways of the sensory nerves and tuning the brain and mind to more subtle, internal stimuli, a remarkable, almost paradoxical result occurs. Although our nervous systems and minds are externally focused, their ability to make accurate contact with the actuality of life is limited. This limitation is not necessary, but is almost inevitable. It results from the activity of memory, and the utilization of habit to streamline responses and navigate the world. The brain learns to interpret the present in terms of the past so as to better understand it. What this leads to for most of us is that we no longer look out on the world with fresh eyes, like a child does. Our perceptions are jaded. We think we know what is coming. We take things for granted. Yoga is designed to overcome this. The internalizing of awareness that yoga brings makes us aware of these habituated patterns of assumption, expectation, and prejudice with which we filter the naked brilliance of the world into safe, familiar shadows of itself. Then, having seen this mechanism, both what it is doing and how it is doing it, we can let go of it. We begin to bring a more childlike quality to our interactions with the world. We rediscover the curiosity, amazement, and joy that we lost somewhere on the road from childhood. We can encounter and enjoy the world more fully, as it actually is. This is the paradox. Simply by developing the capacity to turn the nerves and mind inward the ability to see outward more clearly is developed.

The perceptual and motor enhancement that yoga brings to our nervous system has other, more directly practical benefits. It makes both our perceptions and our actions more accurate. This makes all and any of our daily activities more efficient. We gauge distance, space, color, form, etc. with greater accuracy. We move our muscles more freely, more efficiently. We can hammer a nail, build a shed, mix concrete, lay a path, change a lightbulb or a nappy, lift a pot, clean a child, memorize lines, recall information, calculate a cashflow balance, gauge a client all more easily, more efficiently, and more enjoyably. Having a body and mind that function well, easily and effortlessly brings a simple, priceless delight to the simplest and most mundane activity. Anything at all can be as delightful and rewarding as watching your child take its first step, jumping a hedge on a thoroughbred, scoring a goal in the last minute of a cup final, or whatever it is that gives you the thrill and satisfaction being alive. Yoga not only makes this very clear, but possible, moment by moment.

YOGA AND LIFE

Yoga is not an escape from life. It is not a way of avoiding the challenges and difficulties of life. It is a way of learning how to live life more deeply, more fully, more truly. A way of learning how to enjoy life. A way of enriching it very simply and very easily. It is not a religion, it is a spiritual practice. This means that it does not ask nor require you to take on board any beliefs whatsoever. This not only includes religious beliefs, but also other beliefs and belief systems. You can bring whatever beliefs and belief systems that you like to yoga. It may be that they will change in the face of your experience, but that is for you to decide.

Neither do you have to give up any aspect of your lifestyle. No job or career path precludes yoga. Again though, you may find that your practice of yoga, by bringing you closer to yourself, causes you to re-evaluate your career. We often live our lives from values we have unconsciously absorbed somewhere along the way. Yoga can allow us to discover our own values in keeping with our own character, our own dreams, desires, and direction. This may then lead to a change of direction in work. It could also lead to other kinds of changes too.

One area yoga often makes a big impact is sex. Many people think that yoga and sex are at opposite ends of the spectrum of life. This could hardly be further from the truth. Yoga is internalized sex. Yoga is a very physical, sensual practice; we spend a lot of time focusing on our bodies and how they feel. We are also encountering, focusing, and rechanelling the very energies that we express in sex. Yoga gives us a lot of vitality—energy. This energy is available for any activity, including sex. It also gives us stamina and sensitivity, both of which contribute to our enjoyment of sex. Many women find that practicing yoga can make them feel very sexy. There is no doubt that being and feeling comfortable with one's body and oneself is an appealing,

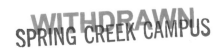

sexy quality. Some people find that their increased general energy level spills over into an increase in sexual appetite and stamina. This is a healthy and encouraging sign. It should not be regarded as unspiritual or unhealthy.

Changes also often occur in people's diet. This happens quite naturally. Yoga makes you more sensitive to your body. This makes you more aware of how foods affect you. You may start to realize that certain foods do not really agree with you. You will then find that you eat them less and less. You do not need to force this. Nor do you need to impose any conceptualized notions of what you should eat on yourself. Certainly you do not need to be vegetarian to practice yoga, although most people who practice yoga find that their desire for meat and other animal products lessens. But this does not happen to everybody. You may also find less need and interest in stimulants. When you give up certain stimulants, like tobacco, coffee, and tea, you can experience unpleasant withdrawal symptoms, which include strong headaches, nausea, fatigue, and nervousness. These will pass after a while.

Yoga is about making friends with life and with yourself. It is not about making life harder by surrounding yourself with a new and fictional code of rights and wrongs, shoulds and shouldn'ts. There is no lifestyle, no occupation, no situation that cannot be greatly enhanced by yoga. Yoga is not something that should be set apart from one's life. Rather it should become the tap-root from which the other aspects of your life are nourished and regenerated.

PART TWO

Method

The method of yoga is very simple. It involves combining the use of structure, movement, breathing, energy, and awareness into a single, unified whole. Each one of these five elements underlies the five classical techniques of *asana*, *vinyasa*, *bandha*, *pranayama* and *drushti*. Together they form a single dynamic unity that renders the practice of yoga as simple as it is powerful, as safe as it is effective, as enjoyable as it is rewarding. There is nothing sloppy or hit and miss about yoga. It is important to have a clear, practical overview of how it works, and how to go about it. Yoga can be divided into the body part—what to do—and the mind part—how to go about it. The body part, the technical aspect of yoga practice, is dealt with in detail in the following sections. It is an exact process. However, when it is clearly understood it is very, very simple. The precision that the technique requires is understood and welcomed by the body on an unconscious level. There is no need for a profound study of anatomy or physiology. You can get help for this part of the practice from any competent and well-trained teacher.

The mind part is more subtle, and more evasive. Our motivation and attitude totally color the way that we implement the technique. They also completely determine the exact nature of its psychological impact. It is therefore important that our motivation and attitude are clarified. To a certain extent our motive for practicing is fixed, but we can modify it. The closer our motivation is to simply **wishing** to find out just exactly what is happening, just exactly what we **are capable** of and who exactly we are, the more fruitful our practice will be. Any preconceived notion of what we want to get out of the practice will predetermine and limit its effect. We will perhaps achieve it, but we will never know what we did not experience because we were not open. Attitude also determines outcome. The most fruitful attitude is one of honesty combined with sensitivity. This means being willing to listen continuously to the feedback the body and mind give during practice. To listen and respond to it: to develop an ongoing relationship with the body/mind that is based on trust and respect. Your body and mind are your most valuable assets. Respect and nurture them and they will repay you over and over again. Mistreat them and they will dog your every step. Respecting the body/mind means not trying to impose on them. Not trying to force the body to become stronger or more flexible. Not trying to force the mind to become more focused or empty. Imposing on the body will lead to pain, exhaustion and anger. Imposing on the mind brings frustration, conflict and confusion. Both kinds of imposition are acts of aggression, of violence against yourself. Practice should be an open inquiry carried out with honesty and sensitivity. Then it will be able to bear its richest fruit—the flowering of our inner nature that transforms our lives into precious jewels beyond price.

Method

STRUCTURE IN YOGA

Yoga postures are very definite shapes. They each have an intrinsic structural integrity. This structural integrity is what gives the postures the deep stillness that both body and mind require for yoga to do its work. Each posture differs from the others in the exact nature of that structure. Yet each one builds its specific structure according to the same structural principles. These are, of course, based on the fundamental laws of physics, anatomy and movement that operate below the threshold of awareness. However, it is not necessary to have a specialist's grasp of these principles to do yoga safely and effectively. It is enough to understand their practical implications in terms of how to move, arrange, and adjust the body.

1. The most important point to grasp is that all postures are supported on the floor, or the mat. That part of the body in contact with the floor or mat is the foundation. The way that the foundation is activated against the floor is crucial. Every other structural consideration depends and rests upon it. The foundation should bear the weight of the body **actively** and **evenly**. *Active support* for the body means that the foundation resists against the floor to create an equal and opposite momentum upwards. It is a little like putting down roots in order to grow a trunk and branches. The force of gravity is utilized to ground the body so that it becomes stable and secure. From this secure stability the rest of the body can safely arrange itself into the required shape, however exotic or unfamiliar. Without the security of a stable foundation it will be more difficult to establish the postures with integrity and safety. It will also be more difficult to feel comfortable, and to relax in those postures that can be established. *Even support* from the foundation means that the weight of the body is carried evenly across the whole foundation. This extremely simple point is only too often overlooked. If this is established postures become not only much easier

and simpler to achieve but also much safer and far more effective. This means that when standing on two feet the weight is distributed evenly between them. It also means that it is distributed equally between the heels and the balls of the feet; likewise between the inner and outer edges of the feet. This will necessarily mean that the inner edge of one foot has the same weight on it as the outer edge of the other—and that the ball of the big left toe has the same weight as the ball of the little right toe. It should be noted that the toes are not included in this equation, except for the balls of the toes, which can be treated as part of the ball of the foot. When standing on one leg the same rationale applies. When the feet share the weight with the hands it is the same. It is also exactly the same when sitting on the floor. There are hundreds of floor postures. The parts of the body making up the foundation vary. Nevertheless the foundation always expresses the same principle of even and equal distribution of weight and action. It may be the backs of the legs and buttockbones; it may be the shoulders, elbows, and back of the head; it may be the head, elbows, and forearms; it may be the back of one leg, one foot, and the buttockbones. The same principle always applies.

2. The second key point is that the core of the body should always be soft, open and passive. There should never be tension in the pelvic floor, the abdomen, the throat, the jaw, the forehead, the eyes, the ears, or the brain. The quality of the core of the body is vital. It must be continuously checked and pacified. Tension in the core of the body is deeply entrenched and hard to clear; especially in the brain and the anus. To release this tension requires continual attention. When the core is soft we can relax: the parasympathetic nervous system can take over from the sympathetic. The core of our body is a doorway to our inner nature. While our body is finite and limited, our inner nature is infinite and unlimited. Uniting the two is part of the purpose of yoga.

Then the physical, limited body can be actively supported by the limitlessness of our inner nature. This depends upon a complete absence of tension from the core of the body. Any tension in the core inhibits the flow of nourishment and support from the core to the body, from the unlimited to the limited, from the infinite to the finite.

3. The third point is that the larger anatomical muscles of the outer body are used to create stability and support for the lungs and the core of the body: so that the core of the body can open and draw nourishment from the universe within; so that the lungs can open and draw nourishment from the universe without. The anatomical muscles do this by contraction of their fibers, but it is done in an unfamiliar way. It is not a matter of contracting the central body of the muscle and creating a shortening of the muscle with a bulging center. Rather it is a matter of learning to gently and specifically contract the ends of the muscles, the origin and insertion, while keeping the central part passive. This causes a lengthening and flattening of the central part of the muscle body. It is a process which takes time to learn. Be patient. If the effort you are making to activate the muscles of the limbs and trunk is exhausting you, you are approaching it in the wrong way. The correct way of utilizing contraction in the muscles uses very little effort and energy, and can be sustained throughout the large muscles indefinitely. Rather than the muscles feeling as if they are hardening and bulking, they feel like they are sucking in towards the bone and wrapping themselves inwards.

4. The fourth point is that the lungs should be given space to open. This is a matter of broadening from the ribcrests to the collarbones, while lengthening through the spine. This is simply a matter of enhancing the natural action of the inhalation, which inflates the ribcage from the back and sides to the front and top. This enhancement, however,

should be done continuously, even while exhaling. It is supported by the use of the arms, which are activated by turning the upper arms so that the biceps turn away from the chest. This lengthens the pectoral muscle of the chest and helps to open the top lung.

5.   The fifth key point is that the waist should be long, and the abdomen passive. There are certain exceptions to this, where the body is curled up and the front of the body becomes short, such as in the **Embryo Pose** and the **Fetus Pose**. Keeping the waist long means that the breastbone is kept away from the pubic bones, and the armpits and floating ribs are kept away from the hipbones. The long, vertical muscles of the central abdomen are kept passive. Because the waist is being lengthened these abdominal muscles increase their tone however. This is not a result of contraction in the muscle body. Do not press in, back, or up with your abdominal muscles. This is a common fault that inhibits the opening of the lungs and keeps the core of the body tense.

6.   The sixth point is that the limbs connecting the foundation to the trunk are working. This means that the stability established in the foundation is transmitted to the trunk as a sense of security and safety. Then the trunk will feel able to open, release, and extend more freely without forcefulness.

7.   The last key point is that all body parts are either deliberately working or deliberately relaxed. If a part of the body is passive it is because you want, and have chosen, it to be so. If a part of the body is active it is because you want, and have chosen, it to be so.

All of these points require the conscious, deliberate and precise application of specific lines of force. The combined effect of these lines of force is to

Method

establish stability, comfort, and presence of mind within each posture. These lines of force create an interbalancing network in which each line of force operates with the minimum effort possible. When all the required lines of force are simultaneously activated, each one requires very little effort. They all support and complement each other throughout the three dimensions of the body. Excessive force applied along any particular line will create imbalance and require other excessive lines of force to stabilize it. This results in overworking the posture and can be felt as instability, tension, or rigidity. Whereas when the structural integrity of a posture is established the posture is effortlessly stable, relaxed, and forgiving.

MOVEMENT IN YOGA

Although the stillness of holding the yoga postures indefinitely is unique to yoga the quality of movement is also vital. All movements should be slow, smooth and effortless. There should be no jerking, no force, no hurrying. The key is learning to harmonize the movement of the body with the movement of the lungs. The activity of the motor muscles should be synchronized with the activity of the respiratory muscles. This means that the activity of the anatomical body is being synchronized with the activity of the physiological body. It is important that the physiological body—the lungs—leads and the anatomical body follows. The breath should not be forced to follow the body. In yoga we are learning to activate from within. To give the deep and the subtle precedence over the superficial and the obvious.

What this means is that any and every movement is linked to either an inhalation or an exhalation. When the inhalation or exhalation begins, so does the movement. The movement ends when the inhalation or exhalation does. Not before and not after. The next movement then follows the next phase of the breath, and so on, until the posture is established. Knowing whether to make a movement on the inhalation or on the exhalation is very simple. If the front of the body is opening, inhale. If it is closing, exhale. This is obvious really and can be tested in practice. The same principle applies when leaving a posture. This means that each posture is both established and released step-by-step. Each step of both the entry and exit is synchronized exactly with either an inhalation or an exhalation.

Exactly what makes up a movement is somewhat predetermined and somewhat arbitrary. To begin with it is best to simplify and use many steps, each one composed of a single action. As you progress and become more familiar and comfortable with the supporting actions that constitute the movements

Method

that take you in and out of postures, you can blend different actions together into more comprehensive steps. Each designated step should still be synchronized to either an inhalation or an exhalation. When the lungs are not moving, the body should not be moving. When the body is moving it should be because the lungs are moving. A step, then, is an action, or group of actions taken together, executed on one phase of the breath. The more steps you use the longer it will take to establish the posture, and the slower both your body and mind will be working. The fewer steps you use the quicker the postures will be established, but your body and mind may be being rushed and the result may be a posture that is neither stable nor fruitful.

Dividing the process of entering and leaving postures into simple actions and movements is very important. It not only slows body and mind down, encouraging softness, openness and sensitivity, it also means that there is more chance of establishing the postures more fully, deeply, and effectively. Also that you will become aware of any limitations or restrictions in your body's capacity, and can respect and accommodate them without trying aggressively to impose the posture on them.

Synchronizing actions or movements exactly with the breath is also vital. This is not just a matter of harmonizing the activities of the anatomical and physiological bodies. It is also a question of harmonizing the activity of the mind with that of the body as a whole. To exactly synchronize the raising of the arms with the inhalation, and the lowering of the arms with the exhalation, requires complete attentiveness. It requires that the activity of the body be fully supported by the presence of the mind. If the mind starts to wander, synchronization will not be complete. If the mind is not brought to bear on the body then the fruitfulness of the practice will be diminished considerably. Silence is brought to the mind through establishing stillness in the body, and effortlessness in its moving from stillness to stillness. The body is the doorway to the mind and the breath is the threshold. If the mind is not fully present in the activity of the body, this inattentiveness can allow insensitivity, aggression, and violence to enter the practice and diminish it.

When the movement of the body is fully synchronized with the breath then the whole body is functioning as one, as an integrated whole. This gives the movements of a posture an effortlessness that makes it both more easy and more enjoyable. At the same time less physical energy is used and therefore the practice can continue for longer. This can be easily experienced by standing upright and allowing the arms to rise up above the head and down again to the sides in time with breath. This is moving from **Standing Pose** to **Mountain Pose** and back again. When exact synchronization is established, the arms rise and descend on the power of the breath; very little physical effort is required.

Movement synchronized with the breath acquires an effortless fluidity reminiscent of the movement of Tai Chi. This fluidity is important. It calms and soothes the mind and nerves, and enhances sensitivity. All movements should embody the fluid effortlessness of water flowing. They should not be sudden, harsh, jerky, or forced. There should be an easy, pleasing feeling to the movements that we make in yoga. This is why we move step by clear step into the postures and out again—so that there is no forcefulness, no hurry, no compromise. This does not mean, however, that our movements should always take the line of least resistance, and avoid any blocks or hindrances in the body's structure. Rather the soft fluidity of our movement reveals blocks in our body and allows us to challenge them, by gently and sensitively sustaining the direction of movement until, eventually, the block is dissolved.

This fluidity of movement into and out of the postures is mirrored in the overall continuity of the practice. This means that once we start we do not

Method

stop. This does not mean that we do not stop moving. We become still holding the postures, but this is only an external inactivity. Within the stillness of the structure the internal dynamic that sustains the integrity of the posture continues. This internal dynamic is like a continual flow of water in a fountain. It gives shape to the posture but in a dynamic, vibrant way. Then the postures do not become rigid, but are alive and radiant. When we leave a posture, we do not drop our awareness of our body, our internalization, our presence of mind. We bring these step-by-step into the next posture. In this way our presence of mind, internalization and awareness deepen and stabilize from posture to posture. This does not and cannot happen if we stop to rest between postures. Then the mind is almost guaranteed to wander. The postures should be threaded together in a single dynamic but effortless continuum. Then the practice of the postures begins to be meditation in action.

ENERGY IN YOGA

Yoga is a dynamic practice. It is not just a question of moving the body into weird and wonderful shapes. These shapes, by the nature of their innate integrity, are charged with a highly vibrant radiance. They are energized from within. This energy radiates outwards, filling the whole body with a palpable and visible charge that shimmers out of the skin. A posture energized in this way looks and feels quite different from one that is not. Without this charge a pose does not truly become a yoga posture.

Going deeply into a yoga posture does not mean increasing the stretch or amount of movement. It means increasing this charge so that the whole body begins to radiate a luminous potency that is far more striking than extreme movement. Going deeper into a yoga posture does not require that we push at the limits of our flexibility. Instead we just allow the positioning of the various body parts to challenge our muscles and joints gently. Then we activate the inner charge that takes us deeper into the posture. This will only bring about more movement if that extra movement is naturally available to the body. If it is not, it will not. If we have pushed ourselves too far we will be pulled back. Then, while we hold the posture with this inner charge the body's capacity to move is gently and effortlessly increased as a result. We gain a little movement, a little opening, but we have not pushed for it. We have allowed it to happen as a result of natural inner forces that operate according to their own innate parameters.

This is known as cultivating the edge. The edge of a posture is where we are when we are at the very limit of our safe possibility. It is only if we go to the edge that we grow, that our capacity develops. We do not have to force the edge. It is natural for anything that is alive to grow, to develop its capacity. This does not have to be enforced. Our capacity for movement has virtually no limit. To develop it we have only to use fully what we have, and simply

Method

by doing so, we will have more. Nothing more required. Just use what you have fully and you will find that the next time you have more. If however you are greedy, and use the force of aggression to push the body past its limits, the body will put up resistance. You may hurt yourself, you may suddenly become stiffer, you may become frustrated and angry. All because you are bringing to your practice the wrong attitude. Instead of coming with an attitude of open inquiry you come with aggressive intent. The aggression of this narrow-minded intent is amplified by your practice and manifested into tightness, hardness, frustration, and anger. Then the whole point of yoga is lost.

This internal charge that radiates the whole body is always brought about in the same way. It is a subtle muscular mechanism involving smaller muscles of the trunk. It has three aspects: a lifting, a broadening, and a sealing. It is usually initiated just before going into a posture and then clarified and deepened continuously on each inhalation when in a posture.

The first aspect is a lifting of the ribcage from behind and above using the muscles that open the ribcage on inhalation. While this is easiest to do while inhaling, the muscular action can be sustained even during exhalation. In fact this muscular action is maintained almost continuously throughout yoga practice if possible. This action not only lifts the ribcage but broadens the top chest too. This makes the skin on the front, top, and back chest stretch and come alive.

The second aspect is a broadening of the ribcrests. This is achieved by allowing the floating ribs to expand outwards, like the wings of an eagle, so that the upper abdomen broadens and expands. This is again easiest to do on inhalation but can and should be maintained during exhalation. Combined with the upper lifting action, this seals the skin of the floating ribs downwards and in, as if tucking the liver and stomach in under the ribs.

The action is completed by the third aspect: a sealing of the lower abdomen. This involves making the pubic abdomen flatten, by contracting its edges gently while keeping the central area passive. This has the combined effect of drawing the sacrum into the pelvis, sucking the perineum and anus into the pelvic cavity, and anchoring the diaphragm and ribs as they lift.

These three aspects are really part of a single dynamic. Although the three can be isolated from each other they are always then only a shadow of what they can be when they function together. Together they lift and broaden the chest, open the lungs, lengthen the waist and abdomen, lengthen the lumbar and thoracic spine, suck the solar plexus in, stabilize the lower abdomen, and suck the sacrum and the pelvic floor in. At the same time they bring a strong charge into both the ribcage and the abdomen. The skin is stretched and becomes highly sensitive, stimulating its nerve receptors. All as a result of what is soon experienced and activated as a single opening action in the trunk!

What is felt very clearly is the strong active charge in the chest, a strong passive charge in the abdomen, and the solar plexus and perineum sucking in. What can just as clearly be seen is the lengthening of the spine and the stabilizing of the pelvis, especially the sacrum. What can also be seen and felt is a strong upwards momentum from deep inside. At the same time there is a complementary downwards momentum, which can be seen and felt in the movement of the skin, and the tucking in and down of the shoulderblades and floating ribs. The upper abdomen does not puff out at the end of the inhalation. Instead the inhalation is brought into the top chest by the opening of the top ribs. The ribcage as a whole is not thrust forward, the abdominal muscles are not tightened, nor are they pushed back, in, or up.

Method

Altogether what is experienced is a spirallic charge in the trunk. A charge that rises upward and outward from deep inside while sealing downward and inward on the outside. This spirallic dynamic is then extended out into the whole body, through the arms and legs into the hands and feet. This unifies the whole body into a single energetic continuum which has its source deep in the core of the body. This charge is felt in the arms by opposing the upper and lower arms so that they twist at the elbow like a rope and become stronger and longer. The same happens in the legs, though it is more difficult to establish. The hands and feet more clearly reflect the structural and energetic dynamic of the trunk. Like the chest, the balls of the feet and the base of the fingers broaden. Like the abdomen the center of the foot and palm become more hollow. A strong charge is then felt flowing out from the core to the fingers and toes and back again. This charge gives the postures their radiance and their power. It is a charge that is carried along spirallic lines of force that irradiate the body and support the lines of force of the postures' structure. These structural lines of force also activate spirallically and further enhance the single energetic continuum of the body in all of the postures.

BREATHING IN YOGA

Breath is the very basis of our life. We can go many days without food; a few without water, but it takes only a matter of seconds without air and the brain is seriously damaged. Yet how many of us ever even think about our breath? We take it so much for granted. Yet there is perhaps nothing else in life that can give us so much for so little. Paying attention to the breath is at the root of most realistic schools of meditation. Learning to remain attentive to it can yield the highest spiritual fruit. The Buddha declared that it is one of the few techniques able to deliver mankind from the snare of suffering. He himself used meditative breathing to that end.

In yoga the breath is given great importance. However there are two different approaches to using the breath. There is the Classical approach, defined by Patanjali, who is regarded as the father of yoga, and the modern approach defined by medieval Hatha Yoga texts. They are quite different from each other: both in method and in effect. It is very important to be able to distinguish between them for the safe and effective practice of yoga. In essence, the Classical approach is based on surrender, while the medieval approach is based on control. The former leads to a pacification of the neurotic tendencies of the mind, while the latter feeds on them. The former leads to what Patanjali describes as "the vision of discernment," which means being able to see things as they truly are, without the distortion of personal projection. The latter is said to lead to immunity to suffering and death. Anyone who thinks that yoga is going to remove death and suffering from their lives is walking a razor's edge. Life and death, personality and suffering are inseparable. Who would be rid of one will be rid of the other.

Yoga is not about hiding or escaping from reality. Quite the reverse. It is about seeing through the conditioned projections of our personal reality, and making contact with the actual reality of what exists independent of our perceptions. This is no simple thing. Our attachment to our conditioned projections: our beliefs, assumptions, knowledge, opinions, and prejudices is deep and persuasive. It is the "safe" ground upon which we walk and live. However, it is false ground. What is more, it is full of the seeds of unnecessary suffering. Yoga, and any genuine spiritual training, is a means for relieving us of the false perspective of our personal reality, leaving us in direct contact with the naked brilliance of that which actually is. This is available through the so-called "vision of discernment."

The way that we use the breath is a key to this process. Therefore awareness of the breath is cultivated from the start of yoga practice. This begins with the simple mechanism of harnessing the movements of our body to the flow of our breath. This immediately brings the breath into sharp focus, slows it down spontaneously, and emphasizes its importance. The postures themselves, by the way that they work on the body and affect the breath, further enhance our awareness of the flow and quality of our breathing. Other than this we do not work directly on the breath. It is left to flow freely within the context of our activity. The combination of the anatomical impact of the postures and the presence of our awareness transforms the flow of our breathing. This is enough. We do not need to impose on our breathing. We do not try to make it slow. It slows down by itself. We do not try to make it deep. It deepens naturally as the ribcage opens from the posture work. We do not need to try to make it smooth. It becomes smoother as a result of our attentiveness and as our minds become more stable, more concentrated through the practice of the postures.

The energetics of the yoga postures, by which a charge of vitality is brought into the whole body, have a profound impact on our breathing. Once again, however, we do not have to work directly on the breath to bring this about. By lifting, broadening, and opening the ribcage, and by stabilizing the abdomen and diaphragm, the spirallic charge we bring to the trunk enhances the flow, depth, and speed of our breathing. This is a natural process. Furthermore these subtle anatomical adjustments that we make in the trunk also affect the throat. The throat changes its shape and dimensions. It narrows at the top and opens at the bottom. This slows the breath down and brings it into contact with the throat so it makes a sound. When there is no imposition this sound is soft, smooth, and soothing. This way of breathing is known as the "Breath of Tranquillity." It acts as a mantra on the mind—soothing, quieting, and internalizing it.

When we are moving in and out of the postures we synchronize our activity with our breathing. When we are in the postures we do so too. Every time we inhale we deepen the energetic charge in the body, by clarifying the activity of the trunk. Every time we exhale we surrender the spine to the core, allowing them to rid themselves of all imposition and tension. Using the breath in this way allows us to go deeper into a posture. This deepening comes about without effort, without force, simply by amplifying the rhythm of the breath. The spine softens on the exhalation and lengthens on the inhalation. At the same time the nervous system is pacified, the brain rested, and the mind emptied.

Observation of the quality of our breathing can be used as an accurate gauge of our practice. Whether it is soft or hard, quiet or loud, smooth or rough, fluid or jerky, this tells us where we are. Our breathing should be (as far as possible) soft, quiet, smooth, and fluid. Not because we are trying to make it be so, but because of the way that we are using our body and our mind. If our breathing is not—if it is hard, loud, rough, or jerky—this might be because we are coming up against innate tension which is resisting our challenge. This is unavoidable. But as our practice matures it should happen less and less. As we open more and more to a given posture our breath becomes more and more harmonious within it. Then as we progress

Method

to more difficult postures our breath is once again challenged. Our breathing can also become hard, loud, rough, or jerky because we are being aggressive—trying to force our way further into a posture; seeing it only in terms of quantity of movement. This should be avoided. In either case simply bringing the attention to the breath can center us. In the first case it can help to dissolve the resistance. In the second it can help to draw us out of our aggression.

The breath, then, is a vital key to the effectiveness of our practice. Our main concern should be to release it from the restrictive tensions that have been imposed upon it by life. We should not allow our practice to add to those impositions. Rather than doing anything with the breath on a physical level, our practice is to simply feel it clearly, directly, and continuously. This, in combination with the energizing, grounding, opening, centering, and balancing effect of the postures, will transform our breathing into a source of vitality, clarity, and tranquillity.

AWARENESS IN YOGA

Yoga is often represented as a form of exercise. It is much more than that. It is also sometimes represented as a form of religious ritual. Again, it is far more than that. It is even sometimes represented as a religion. Yet again, it is far more than that. It is too comprehensive and fundamental to be easily categorized in words. To be understood it must be practiced; to be well understood it must be practiced for a lifetime. What is very quickly clear, however, is that even though emphasis is given to moving the body into stillness, it has a huge impact on the mind.

Part of this impact occurs spontaneously. Simply as a result of releasing tension from the body, the mind is also released from its restrictive modes and patterns. Just as we can use the body to make new, refreshing, and invigorating movements we can use the mind in new, inspiring, and revealing ways. But the precision and comprehensiveness of the yoga postures requires a very definite contribution from the mind. The mind must be involved in the physical process of the postures if they are to establish their innate integrity.

The application of the spirallic lines of force that make up the inner actions and adjustments of the postures depend on mental attentiveness. Initially this is actually the major stumbling block to mastering the postures. How to use the mind in a new way? The mind is used to moving outward. It is used to being met by intense, changing and often juicy stimuli. It is used to being fairly passive, receiving the continuous rush of impressions the world gives off. It is used to a linear, sequential mode of perception. In yoga this is all turned around. The mind turns inward. It goes to meet subtle, static, and unrewarding stimuli. It must become active, deliberate, focused. It must develop a panoramic, holistic awareness.

Method

This is a difficult challenge for our habitual, conditioned minds to overcome. However, the physicality of the postures and the clear and simple challenge they represent harnesses the vagrant and unstable tendencies of the mind and puts them to work. The mind must and does learn to constrain its wandering within the structure of the body. It must also learn to use its creativity to make something come about, rather than simply to be pulled and pushed from this to that and round again. It is helped in this by the immediate impact of the postures on the mind: as the postures free the mind from its habit patterns, the mind becomes more receptive, more open, and more adaptable.

Establishing the various spirallic lines of force in a posture challenges and encourages the mind to utilize, develop, and refine various qualities. It requires concentration, attentiveness, clarity, subtlety, and openness. These quickly develop. But if the postures are performed absent-mindedly, or without concern for their inner integrity, they do not.

Only too often in life the mind is not really involved in the activity of the body. The plates are washed by the autopilot while the mind is in Bermuda. The car is driven by the body while the mind is in cloud-cuckoo-land. This split between mind and body is one of the greatest hindrances to a rich, full, and satisfying life. We often think that happiness, contentment, satisfaction, and joy are given to us by external objects, situations, and circumstances. This is not quite true. Of course, the object, situation, or circumstance is part of the equation. But there is another, more important part. The quality of the mind. We have to want, we have to be open, we have to appreciate the object, situation, or circumstance. If this were not so, if happiness intrinsically resided in the Denver Broncos winning two straight Superbowls or Manchester United winning the treble, then anyone who knew that this had happened would have to be happy. But happiness doesn't lie in events. Happiness resides in the mind. Remember how different the first kiss is from the last. Same person, same action, same ingredients: but a world of difference to you.

It is the quality of our awareness, more than anything else, that determines the quality of an experience. It is not the structure or content of the experience. What brings us the deepest satisfaction, happiness, joy, and contentment is an ongoing quality of clear, direct, and open awareness that in meeting the world naturally brings appreciation, energy, and delight. All situations and circumstances are full of energy, full of possibility. It is only when they do not fit our expectations and desires, only because we therefore do not meet them with clear, direct, and open awareness, that they are, to us, unsatisfying and uninteresting. Other circumstances give us delight and satisfaction simply because we meet them with an awareness that is free from assumption, expectation, and prejudice. This is how the mind of a child works. This is why a child, experiencing exactly the same world as we do, is full of vitality, delight, creativity, and happiness. While we, sadly, no longer are.

Yoga teaches us to be more like a child. Not childish, but childlike. It does so very simply. By demanding the presence of the mind in the subtlety of the postures. By demanding that this presence remains involved for long periods. By demanding that this presence be accurate, without sloppiness. And by providing a very clear feedback process if this presence fades into absent-mindedness—an inability to establish or hold the posture. Just by refining the activity of the body, the capacity of the mind is also and equally refined.

This is a remarkable thing. For the mind itself is incredibly elusive. Some scientists are so baffled that they pretend the mind does not really exist. To try to harness the mind with the mind itself is very difficult. This is what is happening in meditation. In yoga we use the body to harness the mind. By

Method

recalibrating the body we recalibrate the mind. By liberating the body from its restrictions we liberate the mind from its limitations. In yoga the body is the gymnasium in which we train and develop the mind in attentiveness, concentration, subtlety, clarity, and comprehensiveness. All of these qualities are required and cultivated by the postures. All of the these qualities then become characteristics of the mind—characteristics which are then available to any and all of the activities of everyday life.

The body, then, is the mandala on which we cultivate the meditative mind. A mind that is open, sensitive, subtle, stable, and content. In the beginning we find it hard to hold the many internal actions of a posture in our awareness, but as we progress in our practice we learn to do so. If there is any measure by which we can assess our progress, this is it: how much of our body and its activity can we hold in our awareness at once? In the beginning the mind has to skip from place to place, from adjustment to adjustment. Eventually however it learns the trick of comprehensiveness, it develops a capacity for panoramic awareness. Then the mind can hold all of the different actions of a posture in its grip at once. The meditative quality of the postures becomes clear. The physical postures become a spiritual practice. It is then that we are practicing yoga.

BALANCE IN YOGA

Yoga is about balance. Balancing the various parts of the anatomical body. Balancing the various parts of the physiological body. Balancing the various aspects of the nervous system. Balancing the various qualities of the mind. Balancing all the different aspects of our being. Yoga is also about being able to make balance in life. Balancing the various aspects of our life: work, play, study. Balancing our practice with the rest of our lives.

There are five main aspects to the practice of yoga that we need to take into account. By doing this we can make sure that our practice is balanced. That it is nourishing and enriching us. If our practice is unbalanced it can drain, deplete, destabilize, unground, overactivate, or inflate us. These five aspects are: structure, movement, breathing, energy, and awareness. By varying the emphasis we give to each of these aspects of the practice we can change its effect.

43

By focusing on structure we become more grounded. By focusing on movement we become more dynamic. By focusing on breathing we become more relaxed. By focusing on energy we become more vital. By focusing on awareness we become more awake. We can continually change the tone and impact of our practice by varying the emphasis we give to these five elements. This variation can be one that runs through the whole of a single session, or it can be one that changes from posture to posture, or posture group to posture group. The possibilities are endless—which means that no matter what state we are in, what life is asking of us, we can adapt our practice to help.

There are other aspects of our practice that we can vary to introduce more balance within our practice and between our practice and our life. We need to make balance between effort and ease: applying enough effort, but not too much; being relaxed but not compromising structural integrity. We need to introduce balance between power and fluidity: between developing and utilizing the ability to resist gravity and move freely, and not fighting with our blocks. We need to introduce balance between developing strength and developing flexibility. We need to introduce balance between developing muscular stamina by holding the postures for longer times, and cardiovascular stamina by moving dynamically from posture to posture and utilizing repetition. We need to introduce balance between activity and rest: between holding the postures and linking the postures dynamically. We need to introduce balance between action and meditation: between what we are doing and how we are doing it. We need to introduce balance between quantity and quality: between how much we do and how well we do it. We need to introduce balance between the inhalation and the exhalation: in terms of duration, speed, depth, and overall quality. We need to introduce balance between attending to detail and assimilating the whole picture. We need to introduce balance between imposition and complacency, finding the parameters within which we can challenge our resistance. We need to introduce balance between striving and enjoyment: between achievement and pleasure.

Only when all these different complementarities are balanced will yoga be able to nourish us continuously through the unpredictable changes of life.

PART THREE

Practice

There are certain conditions that always apply to the practice of yoga. They help to make sure that your practice is as safe and effective as possible. They should always be conscientiously observed until they become natural and automatic. The guidance which follows covers such matters as:

- when to practice
- practicing on an empty stomach
- what to practice
- the sequence of postures
- learning a posture
- entering a posture
- using the posture instructions
- holding postures
- shaking and tension
- repeating postures
- what to wear
- where to practice
- ventilation
- heating
- sweating
- washing after practicing
- illness
- starting again after a break
- injuries

- shock
- aches
- pain
- physical discharge
- tiredness
- emotional discharge
- pregnancy
- children
- enjoying your yoga.

WHEN TO PRACTICE

Yoga practice can be done at any time the stomach is empty. First thing in the morning is the natural time to stretch and awaken the body. Doing yoga first thing is a great way to start the day with a sparkle. It not only activates the whole body, but gets the mind in gear too. However, after a night's sleep the body is more resistant to stretching than later in the day. Practice in the afternoon or evening has the advantage of using muscles that are already softer from a day's use. It also usually has the added advantage of a more relaxed mind—if the day's jobs and tasks have all been done, the mind can focus more easily on the practice without being disturbed by pressing demands. This especially applies to the **Centering Practice**.

Progress in yoga depends upon regular practice. A little often is more beneficial than a lot occasionally. To feel that you are progressing you should practice at least twice a week. However, your progress will be slow and you might not even realize that it is happening. If you aim to practice six days a week it is likely that you will manage to average four or five times! There are bound to be some days when you just cannot practice whatever your intention so you will rarely be able to fulfill your weekly quota. Don't worry about that. You do not have to practice religiously, every day, in order to progress. In fact it is better to have a rest every now and then. This allows the muscles time to assimilate the lengthening work you have been doing. Too much stretching can cause the muscles to tighten and harden up in resistance to overdoing it. Take it easy. Be gentle on your muscles; be gentle on yourself.

PRACTICE ON AN EMPTY STOMACH

Yoga should always be practiced on an empty stomach. If you have food in your stomach many of the postures, especially inversions, forward bends, and strong twists will be uncomfortable. The best time to practice, from this point of view, is first thing in the morning. Wait until you feel the beginnings of hunger before you start practicing. They will soon fade away and not bother you. Generally speaking about three hours should pass before practicing after a normal meal, and about one hour after a snack. In extreme cases a little liquid nourishment can be taken, such as rice or oat milk, and/or fruit juice.

Dairy milk tends to act as an anesthetic and dull sensitivity. It is therefore not recommended to drink cow's milk before practicing. Indian teachings suggest that dairy foods should be taken in the event of a strong practice. This is a superficial, symptomatic response to the overexcitation of the nervous system due to aggressive or impetuous practice of advanced techniques, such as *Pranayama*. Better by far to avoid impetuosity and aggression and have no need for natural anesthetics.

Make sure you rest for at least 20 minutes after strong postures before eating. This can be done either in **The Big Chill** or a sitting posture, or by just hanging out.

WHAT TO PRACTICE

The variety of practices outlined in Part Four gives you many options for your practice. At least one of them will fit quite naturally into any 15-minute window that you have available during the day.

Best for the mornings are the energizing, grounding, and balancing practices. Best for later in the day are the opening, rejuvenating, and centering practices. The energizing and grounding practices will probably make it hard to sleep if done late at night.

When you have become comfortable with the different postures and their sequences, you may combine them. You may also safely develop your creativity in varying your practice according to your daily needs. This should always be done with an acute sensitivity to your body in order to avoid strain or injury.

You can modify, add, or omit postures, but be careful. Make sure more challenging postures are prepared for by easier ones that open the body in the same way, and followed by postures that compensate for them by working in the opposite way.

SEQUENCING GUIDE

The importance of judicious sequencing cannot be overemphasized. Postures cannot be safely sequenced at random. You must sequence them according to their effect on your body and mind.

- The symmetrical standing postures, when done dynamically, warm up the whole body and bring the mind into gear.
- The asymmetrical standing postures awaken the intelligence of the body, making it sensitive and responsive. They also focus and clarify the mind. They should be used to prepare the body for strong movements of the spine.
- Forward bends quieten and internalize the mind while warming up the spine. They should be prepared for with leg work, either in standing or floor postures such as those at the beginning of the opening sequence.
- Twists soften the muscles of the back, open the sacroiliac joints, and stimulate the lungs. They can be used to relieve hardness in the back muscles.
- Backward bends vitalize the mind and body and challenge the spine deeply. They should be prepared for with standing postures, forward bends, and twists and, if strenuous, compensated for with twists and forward bends.
- Strenuous postures should be prepared for by postures which open muscles and joints gently, and followed by calming, pacifying postures.
- Inverted postures should be prepared for by postures that soften the neck and spine, and open and activate the shoulders.

LEARNING A POSTURE

There are two phases in doing yoga postures. The learning, which is more anatomical in nature, and the doing, which becomes more physiological and mental. The learning phase also has two stages: comprehension and assimilation. Mastering a posture is thus a three-step process. Each step must be understood and supported if the posture is to work fully.

Step 1: Learning or understanding what is required of the body by a posture. This is a combined mental and physical process. The mind must have a clear idea of what is required of the body and the body must develop a clear sense of what is being asked by the mind. This depends initially on having the posture and its step-by-step execution clearly described, as in the **Practice** section of this book. But accurate and clear description is only the beginning. The body has actively to assimilate that information into modes of concrete action, through practice. This means knowing how to apply the various lines of force required to establish and maintain a posture.

Step 2: Once the body knows which combination of lines of force to apply, it can begin to assimilate the impact of these lines of force on the habituated structure of the body. The various lines of force challenge what-ever restrictive blocks of tension may be residing in the muscles. As the lines of force dissolve these blocks the body begins to open, and the posture begins to take shape. When all restrictive blocks that hinder that particular posture are released then the posture has been learned. This takes time.

Step 3: Once a posture has been learned, once it can be held effortlessly, it allows the muscles, nerves, and organs to be nourished by its impact on the physiological systems of the body. At the same time it has an effect on the mind by disassociating our sense of self from the restricted, habituated pat-terns of a lifetime.

ENTERING A POSTURE

Postures should be entered with care and awareness. It is a matter of making small, specific steps to go from where you are to where you end up. Each one of these steps should be synchronized with either an inhalation or an exhalation. When you are tired, looking for clarification, or are new to a posture you can hold a step for one, two, or more whole breaths. Then continue with your step-by-step entry.

A posture involves both movement and action. Movements are the obvious changes you make to the shape of the body. Actions are the smaller, often invisible, components of those movements that stabilize, clarify, and sustain them. For example turning your feet to enter a standing pose is a movement; broadening the ball of the foot and grounding the heel are component actions. Many actions continue through the different movements that bring you into a posture.

Each step into the posture is made up of a movement, or group of actions that takes you further into it. Which movement or movements you use to constitute a step depends and will vary—your guiding principle should always be to work up through the structure of the body from the foundation. This makes sure that you start with stability and bring that stability with you. How many steps you use depends both on the posture and your familiarity with it. More complex postures require more steps to establish them with stability. So too do simple but more challenging ones. The more steps you use in the beginning the more deeply you will understand a posture. As your body assimilates and opens to the posture you can reduce the number of steps taken. You can also vary the number of steps from practice to practice. You do not reduce the number of steps by dropping certain actions or movements. Instead you blend together movements or actions that had been separate.

53

Leaving a posture should also be done step by careful step. Usually many less steps are required to leave than to enter, but they are still important. Using steps to leave a posture allows you to leave gracefully and without losing the concentration and stability your presence in, and step-by-step entry to, the posture have given you.

USING THE POSTURE INSTRUCTIONS

You can use the instructions given in Part Four to give you a basis for step-by-step entries into the postures.

Each step has a number. Establish the movements and actions of one step before moving to the next. When moving to the next step, maintain the sustaining actions of the previous steps.

In the beginning you can use a whole breath for each step if you need time to clarify each one. Then you can use an exhalation for one, an inhalation for the next, and so on until you are in the posture. You can also divide each given step into more steps if you want. Later you can combine two adjacent steps and perform them as one. Then you can combine even more adjacent steps and perform them as one.

Reducing the number of steps used to enter a posture should not be hurried. There is nothing to be gained by getting ahead of yourself, and much to be lost. Wait until you are completely familiar with each step before reducing them. This means that you understand what is involved in the step and are able to freely embody it. Eventually you can just use two, or in some cases one step to enter a posture.

HOLDING POSTURES

The yoga postures are meant to be held. Having moved into them step-by-step, we then become still. It is within this stillness that the postures take effect. The muscles learn new relationships, new patterns of action and cooperation.

Initially these new patterns from the various postures combine to release the body from its learned limitations, and promote complete freedom of effective action. Later on these new patterns become matrices of nourishment and regeneration for the whole body and mind.

In all stages of your practice becoming still in the posture is important. In the beginning we are holding the lines of force of the posture to challenge restrictive tension. Later on we are holding the lines of force to promote regeneration, rejuvenation, and vitality. These two stages are, of course, quite different. Nevertheless they form a single continuum. The first stage is required before the second can be reached. The second stage is required for the first to come to fruition. Therefore one does not drop a posture just because it is no longer difficult or challenging. It is only when it is no longer difficult or challenging that it begins to bring real benefit.

It is important to realize that holding a posture in the first stage is quite different from holding it in the second. In the first stage — the therapeutic stage — the challenge presented by tension means that we cannot hold for long before we start to tire. This manifests itself as trembling, wobbling, excessive heat, constricted blood flow, or tightening in the muscles. We must learn to recognize when enough is enough. In the second stage there is no struggle at all: only effortless effort. Here we can stay for as long or as short a time as we wish, but stay a while we must — if the posture is to give us its benefit.

SHAKING AND TENSION

Sometimes the postures can make us shake and this can make us become tense. This shaking can be for a number of reasons. It may be that the posture is not fully grounded. Try to stabilize the posture by regrounding the foundation. If that does not work, it may be that the muscle fibers are not getting enough fuel to maintain their contraction rota within the muscle body. Try to breathe more deeply to supply more oxygen to the muscle cells so they can metabolize more glucose. If this does not work, come slowly and carefully out of the posture. Then go into a more restful posture until you feel ready to try again.

We can become unstable in postures through four different kinds of tiredness: muscular tiredness, cardiovascular tiredness, drowsiness, and sleepiness. Sleepiness should be respected. Lie down in **The Big Chill** and go to sleep. You'll feel much better.

Drowsiness can often be shaken off by the postures of the **Energizing Practice** and also those of the **Grounding Practice**.

Cardiovascular stamina needs to be developed over time. This is a matter of emphasizing the dynamic aspect of moving between and repeating postures.

Muscular stamina is also developed through the practice of holding the postures, especially the standing postures and inversions. However, do not continue to hold a posture if you are shaking excessively or becoming tense.

REPEATING POSTURES

Repetition is fundamental to any learning process. The easiest way to learn is to repeat over and over again. Postures are learned much more easily and enjoyably by repetition than by trying to stay a long time in postures that are not yet stable and comfortable. To stay too long in a posture until muscles are exhausted, nerves are overwhelmed, and shaking or tension sets in is counter-productive. It gives body and mind an unpleasant experience. This then creates resistance to repeating that experience, to repeating that pattern of movement, that posture, in the future. Yoga is not self-mortification. It can and should be continually accompanied by a sense of release, relief, growth, and expansion.

Postures, then, can be repeated more than once. In the beginning this can be done because it is difficult to stay in the postures: by repeating the postures we teach the muscles, nerves, and neural pathways in the brain what is required of them. As they start to accommodate themselves to these requirements through repetition, staying in the posture becomes easier.

This is the same way that infants learn to move and walk. Through hesitant repetition that becomes more and more confident, while a pattern of neuro/muscular action is being learned. When the pattern has been coded in the brain, the action, movement, or posture becomes stable and can be sustained without strain.

We can also use repetition to focus on a specific block. If one leg or hip is tighter than the other we can repeat the posture on that side any number of times.

Repetition can also be used to spice up a practice. By repeating postures dynamically, holding them only for a short time, any practice sequence becomes more invigorating. This is sometimes appropriate and enjoyable.

WHAT TO WEAR

Decency permitting you should wear as little as the temperature and your physique allow, but make sure that those parts of your anatomy that are usually supported remain so. Otherwise the more your skin can breathe the better. If the air is cold however, it is best to wear a thin layer of cotton clothing on the trunk and limbs.

Anything that is worn against the skin should be of a light, natural fiber such as cotton or silk: not wool. Man-made fibers should be avoided against the skin as they desensitize the skin receptors and interfere with your internal feedback processes. Many people find that wearing man-made fabrics anywhere, but especially against the skin, can cause fatigue and lack of clarity.

Whatever is being worn should not be tight: it should not create marks on the skin. This will interfere with the circulation of blood and lymph, and the transmission of nervous impulses in the sensory motor nervous system. Yoga is a process of developing refined and subtle responsiveness to the automatic processes of the body. It is best not to hinder this.

Socks should never be worn, especially when the feet are working against the floor. Even at other times it desensitizes the feet and inhibits their ability to support the activity of the legs, which is vital even when the feet are not on the floor.

WHERE TO PRACTICE

A flat space of six feet by two feet (1.8 meters by 60 centimeters) is all you need to practice yoga. Of course, the more space you have the more comfortable it will feel. However if you do not have a large space available do not be put off practicing in a hallway, bathroom, or small bedroom.

To get a good grip when doing postures that require it, a non-slip yoga mat is a must. The most important requirement is that the ground on which you are working is as flat as possible. If this is not the case structural distortions in the body will occur that will diminish the structural benefits of the postures.

Do not practice in a draught. The contrast between the internal warming effect of the postures and the cold airflow can traumatize the muscles into tightening, and even pulling.

If practicing outside grass provides an adequate surface. Sand is also a usable surface. Rumor has it that the ancient yogis used to practice in the sandy riverbed of the Ganges river. Many postures are made easier thanks to the way that sand gives to the contours of your body. Again, make sure that there is not a cold breeze blowing. If the air is warm you will find the relaxing effect of nature makes your muscles very soft and easy to open. However, do not practice in direct, strong sunlight. This can cause overheating, excess sweating, exhaustion, and headaches.

While mirrors can be useful in gauging how balanced your use is of the body, they are not recommended for regular practice. Looking in the mirror makes it impossible to feel internally with the precision required of the postures. It also tends to cultivate unhelpful tendencies such as vanity, or its opposite.

Although it is pleasant and calming to practice in a quiet place without the sound of traffic or human activity, it is not necessary. In fact it can become addictive to the point of making it impossible to practice without complete silence. This can then become a weak excuse for avoiding practice if your circumstances change.

VENTILATION

If practicing indoors make sure that the room is well ventilated without being draughty. This does not mean that any windows need to be wide open. Just a little crack is enough. Even that may be unnecessary in a large room, or a room in a large, airy house with its door open. A good supply of oxygen is necessary if your muscles are not to become fatigued. A lack of oxygen will make you feel drowsy and uncomfortable. However, too much airflow, even if not as concentrated as a draught, can inhibit the warming effect of the practice.

Make sure that there are no strong smells or scents that might irritate your nostrils, throat, or lungs. These might include cleaning fluids, perfumes, smoke, and even incense. The effect that yoga practice has on your breathing means that any noxious gasses in the air will be taken deep into your lungs. Even incense smoke is harmful to your lungs, despite pleasing your nostrils and mind. Natural scents such as flowers or herbs should not normally cause any problem.

HEATING

Simple observation shows that people who live in a warmer climate tend to be more flexible than those who live in a cold climate. Being an Indian practice, yoga was developed in a very warm climate. Stretching muscles and opening joints is much easier in the warmth. Do not practice in the cold. Cold wintry air can have the same effect as a draught. The contrast it makes with the warming effect of the postures can traumatize your muscles into tightening and even pulling. If your skin feels cold when you are about to start practicing, turn on the heating.

The higher the temperature in which you practice the more readily muscles and other body tissues will open, lengthen and recalibrate. However as the temperature increases and muscles soften, ligaments and tendons become less stable. This can lead to strain and even dislocation in extreme cases. Excessive heat can also cause drowsiness and headache, and bring on a sense of fatigue. Therefore a happy medium must be found by trial and error if you are going to use artificial heating. Remember that during the summer you will need less artificial heat, because your muscles will have a softer residual state.

Beware of creating a room temperature that is much hotter than the outdoor temperature. While this will make your practice easier it may not be as helpful as it feels in the long term. The marked and imposed contrast between your practice temperature and the climatic air temperature can cause strong, reactive muscle hardening when you expose yourself to the colder air. This can especially occur in muscles or muscle groups that have previously been injured or which are very tight.

SWEATING

Yoga is designed to make you sweat. It is known as a fire practice: one in which you purify your body by heat. The heat generated by the postures stimulates cellular detoxification. Creating heat internally stimulates the movement of liquid to the skin. This can include melting fat deposits which often harbor stored toxins. The presence of sweat on the skin functions as a thermal shield. The sweat acts like a wet suit providing insulation against the cooler external air. Then the heat generated in the practice stays inside—softening tissues, opening joints, and flushing out toxins.

Your sweat should be generated by your activity. To bring yourself to a point of sweating you may need to practice more dynamically. This means both connecting the postures into flowing sequences, and activating the whole of the body internally. Just holding the **Staff Pose**, for example, is enough to bring on a sweat if it is done with attention to the muscular adjustments that integrate the posture.

However it is possible to overheat; heat should not be artificially stimulated. Turning up your heating system excessively to make you sweat more has a weakening effect. It causes sweat to drip off the body as part of the heat loss process. To maintain the same level of heat without a static thermal layer of sweat, the body has to work harder than necessary. This can lead to short term exhaustion and long term depletion of energy and vitality.

If you are sweating profusely during your practice you can slow down, insert some cooler resting postures, and make sure you are not pushing for more movement in the postures. However, do not wipe the sweat off your body or face during practice. This will simply cause the body to overwork to replace it. Let it drip and drop. If it is stinging your eyes, just wipe your eyes, not your forehead, and slow down.

CLEANING THE BODY

Yoga practice causes toxic discharge, even when you do not sweat. You will therefore want to bathe after your practice. It is best not to do so too soon. The practice not only brings toxins to the surface, but minerals also. Time must be given for the body to reabsorb them so as not to develop any mineral deficiency. Tradition maintains that it is best to rub the sweat back into your body at the end of your practice so as to ensure no mineral loss. This can be done as you lie down for **The Big Chill**.

Best then to wait half an hour after you have finished your practice to shower or bathe. Always make sure that your water is not too hot. This can also cause mineral depletion and exhaustion.

ILLNESS

Even when bedridden by illness we can still practice yoga. We can use the **Centering Practice** even when lying down. We can also simply stretch the fingers, toes, legs, and arms according to the principles set out in this book. This will help to promote circulation, which is compromised by inactivity.

When ill but not confined to bed, the **Centering Practice** is also beneficial. So too is the **Rejuvenating Practice.** When no longer ill but convalescing, the **Opening Practice** can be introduced.

The use of these three practices will promote recovery provided they are used with sensitivity and honesty. Go slowly, rest when you need to in **The Big Chill**, and do not force anything. Spend plenty of time lying in **The Big Chill** at the beginning of your practice as well as at the end. Wait to use the **Energizing**, **Grounding**, and **Balancing** practices until your use of the other practices has brought you up to par.

If you are experiencing the following conditions please consult a medical professional with an understanding of yoga and a yoga teacher familiar with the therapeutic application of yoga. Yoga done with an understanding of its therapeutic application can benefit these conditions:

- cardiac problems
- cancer
- AIDS
- M.S.
- Chronic fatigue syndrome (M.E.)
- epilepsy
- arthritis
- knee problems
- neck problems.

STARTING AGAIN AFTER A LONG BREAK

When your practice has been displaced by life's pressing demands, do not rush straight back into it. Go slowly. Do not expect to be able to do what you could when last you practiced.

Start first with the **Rejuvenating Practice**, then introduce the **Grounding Practice**, then the **Opening Practice**, then the **Energizing Practice**, and finally the **Balancing Practice**.

Go slowly through the postures, and take many steps to enter each posture. Take time to hold each posture.

INJURIES

Yoga can have a healing effect on old injuries. However this should not be taken for granted. When the body's movement is specifically restricted by the presence of an old injury it is especially important to proceed with caution. Do not push your way into the resistance. Go gently, using the exhalation to bring about softening in the tissues. Stay at your comfortable limit and breathe freely and fully while emphasizing the exhalation.

More recent injuries must also be approached with the same caution. It is important to stay focused on the injured area so that you can respond to the feedback it provides immediately.

Neither old nor recent injuries should be an excuse for not practicing, but they may require that the practice be modified, at least for a while. Neck and knee injuries in particular must be accommodated. Never persist in a posture if you have pain around or in the kneecap, or in the neck. If you cannot release the pain by rearranging yourself in the posture, come out and try to enter it again with a greater awareness of the painful area and how what you are doing is affecting it. If this does not work, pass on to the next posture. If you consistently have a problem with knees or neck, consult a specialist.

68

SHOCK

Old injuries are going to be challenged and released by a yoga practice that is consistent and deep. It is important to be ready for this and how it can feel. Even so, it can still come as something of a shock.

Old injuries will exist as a combination of tight muscles, scar tissue, and restricted movement. As the yoga postures begin to reopen the body the tight muscles of old injuries are loosened, movement begins to return, and scar tissue begins to be activated and stretched. This means that blood flow, as well as movement, will begin to return to the injured area. This will promote both cleansing and regeneration.

Tight muscles, ligaments, and tendons will give and open much more easily than scar tissue. They will therefore tend to open little-by-little without much indication that anything is happening. However, once the muscles and connective tissue have been released, revitalized, and stabilized then the postures begin to work directly on the scar tissue. It has to be broken down and replaced.

Sometimes the breaking down occurs slowly and imperceptibly. Sometimes it doesn't—it happens suddenly and without warning. The scar tissue opens and releases completely and this can be felt as a ripping or tearing sensation. This sensation is usually completely free of pain as these tissues are already dead. However the suddenness, combined with the sensation of tearing, can shock the mind. This shock can cause a reflex tightening action in the nearby muscles that can send them into spasm. This can be painful, but it is not necessary. If you are prepared for this possibility you will recognize it and be able to stay relaxed, so that the release can occur unhindered. Sometimes the shock destabilizes surrounding muscles and you don't have the strength to continue. Lie on your back

Practice

and do some simple movements until your power returns. This tearing sensation can occur more than once in the same place, until the release is complete.

ACHES

Yoga is going to make your muscles ache. Most of our muscles have not been fully used, and have become too short. They ache during yoga because they are being awakened. The muscles are being lengthened back to their optimal length. They are being asked to use their fibers in ways that they are no longer used to. Once the muscle fibers have re-awoken this should stop. Then as you proceed to lengthen the muscles further they will not necessarily ache as you do so, provided you do so slowly but surely, little-by-little, day-by-day. If you push past your limits the muscle will ache and then tighten in response. If you stop practicing, when you start again you will probably again have to go through a temporary aching period. Over time this period gets shorter and shorter.

A muscle that aches aches exactly in proportion with your use of the muscle. As you go deeper into the stretch the ache increases. If you lessen the stretch the ache begins to fade. As soon as you change the posture the ache stops. If it continues it is because you ignored the signals, pushed past the limit, and strained the muscle. This is not necessary and just leads to muscle tightening, which will produce more aching when it is released.

The best way to deal with muscles that ache the day after a practice is to practice again. Not practicing because they hurt just prolongs the re-awakening process. Each time you start again your muscles will ache, and you will never get to the point where there is no more aching even though muscles are still being lengthened.

Sometimes we have such a strong mental resistance to muscles aching that it feels like pain. We have to learn to distinguish between the activity of the nerves and that of the mind. Then we can know if what the nerves are transmitting is really pain, or actually just effort.

PAIN

Pain, as opposed to aching or shock, is not necessary in yoga. However until our sensitivity, honesty, and responsiveness are perfect we will experience some pain now and then. It may be from pushing into an old injury. It may be from pushing into tight muscles. It may even be by using a muscle the wrong way. There is no need to push. Probe gently with honest sensitivity and you will reach your limit. Reaching your limit naturally extends it. Pushing past it diminishes it.

Whatever the reason your response should be the same. Do not sustain the actions that bring pain. Pain is the body's warning signal that cells are under strain to the point of harm. This is always the case. Even if it only results in minor muscle tearing, pain will bring with it a protective muscular tightening that is the opposite of what you are looking for. Just stop. Back off and resume the posture with a greater concern for sensitivity and awareness than for movement—for quality rather than quantity.

You should respond *immediately* to both knee and neck pain by releasing the action or movement that brought it on. There should be no hesitation over this: you only have one neck, and only one knee for each leg. You will deeply regret it if you lose the free use of any of them. Many Western knees are not and never will be ready for the full lotus position. Trying to force the full lotus on yourself can result in permanent damage to the knee that will not only prevent full lotus but many other movements that your life requires, let alone your practice. Nor should you be in a hurry to do the headstand or the shoulderstand. Both require an intelligence in the body that allows the whole body to resist gravity, rather than the effect of gravity being carried by the neck alone. This intelligence is awakened through repetitive practice of more basic postures, especially the standing postures.

PHYSICAL DISCHARGE

Yoga is a therapeutic practice. It works deeply into the body. This is not only a structural process, but a cleansing one also. Every cell in the body can be subject to increased circulation and internal massage by the practice of yoga. This leads to a very efficient clean out of residual waste products and accumulated toxins. These toxic residues are brought initially into the blood. From there they can leave the body in a number of ways.

The simplest way is in the case of gaseous wastes that are discharged through the lungs on the exhalation. This process can give the exhalation a potent aroma. This should pass soon after the practice is over.

Toxins can be discharged naturally through urine and feces. This can give them both unusual colors and/or texture. After a while this will pass. Toxins can also be discharged through the skin: this can be as a skin rash, pimples, boils, or temporary discoloration and change of texture.

73

Other physical reactions to the presence of toxins in the blood include headaches, fatigue, drowsiness, and aching in the joints. All these too should be temporary.

If any of these things happen for a long period, consult an holistic medical practitioner with an understanding of the radical power of food. It may be that something you are eating on a regular basis is not agreeing with you. It may also be that you are overexerting yourself and disturbing the natural balance of your organs. Be careful.

TIREDNESS

Many people experience deep tiredness after beginning to practice yoga. Sometimes they mistake this to be a sign that the yoga is exhausting them. This is rarely the case.

The fact is that most of us lead lives that do not allow enough rest. We are under so much pressure and suffer so much stress to get on that we are in a state of permanent semi-exhaustion. In order that this state does not hinder our productivity, we mask it with a wide variety of stimulants. Some people are addicted to coffee, some to tea, others to sugar. Some are addicted to alcohol, some to cocaine. Some are addicted to a mix of all or some of these substances, all of which are drugs, even the ones that masquerade as foodstuffs.

When we do yoga it relaxes us. The sympathetic nervous system that has been kept turned on by life and drugs, turns off, and the parasympathetic system is activated. As the whole of our system slows down and begins to regenerate itself, we are no longer insensitive to our state of residual tiredness. Simply practicing yoga, because it relaxes us and nourishes the parasympathetic nervous system, will help us to recover from this state. Yoga also helps us to be aware of the harmful coping strategies we use in life, and can help us to develop more beneficial ones: perhaps the best of all these being the regular practice of yoga!

EMOTIONAL DISCHARGE

Yoga is a profound practice. It works deeply into the mind. Many emotional and psychological blocks can be released by yoga, giving you the opportunity to resolve them. This does not happen by itself. In order to resolve emotional and psychological releases a period of silent stillness is necessary at the end of your practice. This can be while sitting in **Easy Pose** or **Adepts Pose**, or in **The Big Chill**. In this silent stillness the released blocks can be resolved into the tranquil openness of your awareness. This may or may not involve memory of the original cause of the block. What is more important is that you give the heart and mind time to establish themselves in harmony before engaging with the hurly burly of the world again.

If you do not give yourself this space for psychological assimilation then you might re-enter the world off-center. You may feel impatient, angry, frustrated, melancholic, confused, resentful, anxious, timid, uncertain, or whatever. This is usually a sign that your practice has worked deeply enough to promote release, but has not been spacious enough to permit resolution. If you can, just take the time to sit or lie in silent stillness, and allow your awareness to clarify itself as in the **Centering Practice**, without resisting the coming and going of your thoughts and feelings.

However it may be that these feelings are present because of impetuous or shallow practice. Anger, irritation, frustration, and impatience can all result from an aggressive approach to practice. A half-hearted practice, undermined by absent-mindedness, can produce melancholic feelings, timidity, anxiety, resentment, and confusion.

PREGNANCY

Yoga is the perfect practice for pregnancy. It is a gentle, comprehensive practice that develops and maintains fitness, flexibility, tranquillity, and vitality. It is especially beneficial for its effects on respiration, circulation, and digestion. These benefits for the mother lead to improved nourishment for the baby.

However, no new exercise program should be begun during pregnancy unless under direct supervision. For those already practicing yoga, you should feel free to continue, taking into account the need to modify the practice as the pregnancy develops.

In general, care must be taken with twists and forward bends because of the pressure they can put on the uterus. Strong twists and forward bends should be avoided. No force or pressure should be applied to the abdomen in any way.

The first three months can be precarious for some embryos. Therefore mothers-to-be should take great care not to put themselves through any stress as a result of yoga practice. Practice gently and quietly, with sensitivity to feedback received from body and mind. Many women are especially intuitive during pregnancy and any intuitive feeling to not do something should be respected.

The second three months of pregnancy are less precarious, but the size of the uterus means that certain movements begin to be restricted—especially forward bends. These can be modified, both in leg positioning, by making space, and in the forward movement, which should diminish.

The last three months require even more modifications because of restricted movement. Forward bends can be transformed into sitting postures. Inversions should only be done if you are both completely confident and completely comfortable.

For specific guidance for yoga in pregnancy please consult *Preparing for Birth with Yoga* by Janet Balaskas (published by Element Books).

CHILDREN

Young children love to do yoga. They do it spontaneously, unconsciously. They love to stretch, challenge, and enjoy their bodies. It may be possible to harness this faculty, but it may just as easily be that doing so will inhibit it. It is best to allow children to come to yoga from their own desire and interest. If they do it should be presented as fun. The postures can be related to animals or objects, and doing them can be turned into a game.

Children should not be asked or expected to do the postures with precision. The geometry of the postures is based on the geometry of mature bodies. The relationships between the bones and muscles in an adult body differ from those of children. Those of children are also different at different stages of their development. Just allow children to use their innate faculty for imitation to do the postures that you show them in any way that they feel like. Remember that things that would frighten and hurt you may well neither hurt nor frighten children. Do not impose your fragile limitations on them. Do not teach them to be less than they are, less than they can be.

If you do yoga and have a family it is important both for your relationship with them and for their well-being that you do not make an issue out of your practice. Make sure that it does not become a barrier between you and your family. Integrate your children into your practice and they will not resent it. Cut them off from it and they will resent you also. Yoga is about dissolving divisions, not creating them. Enjoy your family, enjoy your yoga, and you may find you can enjoy your yoga, your family, and yourself all at the same time.

ENJOYING

Yoga can be a very sensual experience; very enjoyable, pleasing, and satisfying. It does not have to be some ascetic self-mortification that we undertake only to improve ourselves, somehow. If you do approach it as something you ought to do, or something that has got to be good for you, it probably won't be. Even though the postures can be challenging, overcoming challenges is not only fun but also empowering.

If approached openly, and with a willingness to enjoy it, you will soon find that yoga becomes one of the delights of your life. Something which you do not because you feel you have to, but because you love to. The more you experience your yoga this way, the more it will also benefit you in mundane, practical ways. Your enjoyment will make you more open, more receptive. You will struggle with your limitations less. Instead you will find how to challenge them acceptingly. Then you will find your body responding more easily and more fully. Your tension will dissolve more readily. Your blocks will release more easily. Your practice will be far more fruitful.

Yoga has a remarkable capacity to open the heart, to rekindle the joy of being alive, and to cultivate an appreciation of all that lives and exists. Life is not a punishment. Nor should yoga be. The innate joy, delight, and wonder that life offers is too often lost to adults. Yoga is a very effective way of recovering that joy, wonder, and delight, but only if it is approached with the open, inquiring, and adventurous spirit of a child.

AN ANATOMY OF YOGA

Each part of the body has its own place and role to play. Only too often life has disturbed this whole. Yoga can help to reintegrate the body if it is done with an awareness of where the various body parts are and how they should relate to each other. In the beginning it may seem a little overwhelming to take account of each part of the body. But it soon becomes quite natural. You will quickly discover that the various body parts have basically the same relationship with each other all the time. It is only by changing the overall shape of the whole body that the momentary and obvious form of these relationships change.

Please try to apply these pointers as you read them so that they make sense.

The Feet

Except on the rare occasions when the whole body is completely relaxed, the feet should always be alive and energized. The most important aspect of this is the ball of the foot. It should be kept broad and open. When standing this involves using the balls of the big toe and little toe to create space between them. When the foot is not against the floor, it involves broadening and extending forward from the center of the ball of the foot. Do not push forward with the ball of the big toe. The heels should also be kept broad, usually by spreading from the inner heel to the outer, so that when standing the four corners of the feet—the balls of big and little toe and the inner and outer heels—all press down equally. Engaging the foot in this way also engages the calf muscles, and supports the legs and the pelvis in the standing postures and forward bends.

The Toes

The toes themselves should be relaxed but alive. When standing only the pad of the big toe engages the floor. The rest of the toes extend lightly along the floor without pressing down or crinkling. When the foot is not against the floor the toes extend lightly out of the ball of the foot, neither pushing forward nor pulling back. There should be no crinkling in the toe tendons, all of which should be long.

The Ankles

The ankles are very important joints. They bear the full weight of the body when standing. Most of us have very little movement left in our ankles. It needs to be re-awakened. The four sides of the ankle joint — inner ankle, outer ankle, front ankle, back ankle — all need to be equally open and engaged. If the inner ankle is closed or dropping, the inner leg and inner spine are not fully supported. If the outer ankle is closed or dropping the outer leg and spine are not fully supported. The ankle transmits the activity of the feet to the legs and pelvis to support the spine.

The Calves

The calves activate correctly when the feet are used properly.

The Knees

The knees are a very vulnerable joint. Never allow pain to stay in the knee joint. Try to adjust your position to relieve it. If this does not work, modify or change your posture. Many sports and other activities, including hill walking and driving, can weaken or damage the knees. In order to protect them from injury in yoga and life two things are vital. The first is that the feet are used properly, especially in the standing postures, so that the load on the knee is also even. If the foot is not working properly the load on the knee can be carried excessively by one part of the knee joint, which can strain and eventually tear ligaments. (This is true in all activities not just yoga.) The second point is that the thighs must also work to take the load off the vulnerable knees.

The Thighs

Most important in protecting the knees are the front thigh muscles. They need to be strong, and they need to be activated whenever the leg is not deliberately relaxed. This means that when the leg is straight, it is straight, and the thigh muscles are fully engaged. The front thigh is engaged by sucking the muscles into the bone—then the kneecap lifts. The front thigh is strengthened by **Chair Pose**. It also develops through correct use in all the postures. When all of the thigh muscles are fully engaged, by sucking them into the bone, and the feet are too, the backs of the knees open and broaden and the four bones at the back of the knee come into line.

The hamstrings are very obvious to most people beginning yoga: they ache. Most of us have tight hamstrings, especially if we play sports. Most of the postures require, and develop, long hamstrings. Be patient. To make sure that the hamstrings are not aching unnecessarily due to overwork, fully engage the front thigh muscles and, if standing, make sure your weight is on the ball of the foot. This also helps in the case of hyperextended knees.

The inner and outer thighs are much harder to access than the front and back. They depend on correct use of the feet, ankles, and knees. When standing in **Standing Pose**, **Mountain Pose**, **Chair Pose**, or **Standing Fold** the inner ankles press against each other and back. This should engage the inner thighs. In **Triangle Pose** lifting the inner ankles and hitting the inner knees outward toward the outer knees engages the inner and outer thighs.

The Pelvic Floor

The pelvic floor should always be soft. There should be no hardness in the anal or urogenital muscles. This is much harder to maintain than it is to establish, but it is very important. Awareness of the quality of the pelvic floor is at the very heart of the effectiveness of yoga. It must be patiently cultivated from the outset. The pelvic floor should also be as spacious as possible. This is mainly activated from the feet and knees. Their correct use creates space and lift in the pelvic floor which can be clearly felt. This helps to maintain awareness and the softness of the pelvic floor.

Buttock Bones

When sitting the buttock bones are part of the foundation. They should both be equally on the floor. Usually we sit to the front of the buttock bones so as not to lean back and round the lower back. When doing forward bends this is especially important, as it helps to initiate the forward movement from the pelvis rather than from the back.

In asymmetrical standing postures the line of the buttock bones is vital and is controlled from the feet via the legs. When the pelvis is not turning forward with the front foot, both buttock bones spiral in towards the

Practice

perineum. When the back hip is brought forward the front buttock bone is kept tucked in and spiraling towards the perineum.

The Sacrum

The sacrum is the top of the tailbone. It is a fusion of vertebrae set into the back of the pelvis. Many people have a distortion in the positioning of the sacrum: it is not aligned properly with the pelvis at the sacroiliac joints. By creating space across the pelvic floor and engaging the pubic abdomen, the sacrum is engaged into the pelvis at the sacroiliac joints. Realignment of the sacrum also results from the correct use of the feet and legs in the standing postures, forward bends, twists, and backward bends.

The Hipbones and the Groins

The hipbones are the top front of the pelvis. They must be kept lifted so that the sacrum and the pelvis are vertical. When they are lifted the groins are lengthened. In the beginning the groins may feel a little tight. They should be kept soft and allowed to move backwards toward the sacrum.

The Pubic Bones and Pubic Abdomen

There are two pubic bones at the bottom front of the pelvis. They should be kept as broad as possible by broadening the pubic abdomen so there is a contraction at the edges by the groins, while the central part is passively stretched and flattened. This draws the sacrum in and protects it. The pubic abdomen is the lowest of the three sections of the abdomen. It lies between the pubic bones and the line between the hipbones, and between the groins.

The Navel and Central Abdomen

The central section of the abdomen has the navel at its middle. The bottom is the line between the hipbones, the top is the floating ribs when the waist is long. When the waist is short the bottom of the floating ribs drops to the hipbones. The central area of the abdomen is allowed to remain passive; so too are the long muscles that run each side of the navel.

The Floating Ribs, Ribcrests, and Upper Abdomen

The floating ribs are the lowest ribs that attach to one another rather than to the breastbone. The ribcrest is the line of floating rib ends that descend down and out in a curve from the breastbone towards the hipbones. The area between the floating ribs is the upper abdomen. It should remain passive and never stick out past the line of the ribcrests. When you breath in the ribcrests should broaden as the floating ribs flare up and out and the upper abdomen broadens and flattens. Do not thrust the ribcrests forward.

The Lumbar Spine

The lumbar spine is at the bottom of the back just above the pelvis. It has much more movement than the rest of the spine, and is therefore more vulnerable to injury. Weakness in the abdomen can lead to a lumbar distortion known as swayback. This is very common. To correct this the pubic abdomen must be engaged as the hipbones and ribcage are lifted, so that the lumbar spine lengthens and draws back away from the abdomen.

The Breastbone and Top Ribs

The breastbone is the vertical bone at the top front of the ribcage. The top ribs are connected to it. They rotate upwards as you breathe in, and down again as you breathe out. The bottom of the breastbone should stay in while the top lifts. The collarbones join the top of the breastbone to the shoulders. They should be kept broad to keep the top front lungs open.

The Thoracic Spine

The top spine is the thoracic spine. It should not be excessively rounded. If it is, effort must be made to move the top vertebrae forward towards the breastbone without thrusting the ribs or breastbone forward.

The Shoulders, Shoulderblades, and Armpits

The shoulders should always be kept relaxed and away from the ears. They should also be kept rolled back, with the shoulderblades dropping down the back. Space for the top back lung to open should be kept between the shoulders. Space for the back lung to open should be kept between the shoulderblades. The armpits lift up away from the hipbones, helping to lift the ribcage, lengthen the abdomen, and lengthen the spine.

The Arms and the Hands

The activity of arms and hands supports the opening of the lungs. Arms should be kept long and alive, with palms broad and fingers long. Make sure you are not overworking and causing strain or tension.

The Neck, Throat, and Jaw

The neck should be kept long and centered, with the throat soft. When turning the head keep it in line so the neck does not shorten on one side. Placing the head symmetrically in the line of the shoulders is vital in inversions. The jaw should be kept relaxed, with the lips closed.

The Brain, Eyes, Ears, and Forehead

The brain should be kept soft. So should the eyes and ears. Feel them softening down into the brain, with the brain softening down the spine into the pelvis. The forehead should be kept relaxed. Watch for this when lifting the head, or looking up.

The Core of the Body

The core of the body runs from the brain down the center of the spine into the perineum at the center of the pelvic floor. It should always be soft, passive, and open—especially the forehead, eyes, ears, jaw, navel, anus, and perineum. *Always* keep the anus and brain passive.

PART FOUR

Postures

THE YOGA POSTURES

The most obvious thing about yoga is the shapes into which the body is placed. These shapes are the context within which yoga takes place. They are not themselves yoga. Many of them can be seen in the everyday activity of young children. Many of them can also be seen in the activity of dancers, gymnasts and acrobats. But yoga is none of these—it is more like the activity of children if anything. Yoga, like childhood, is a process of exploration, discovery, empowerment, and delight. It is a process full of trial and error, excitement, confusion, and joy. Just as the actions of a child may resemble those of an adult but have a very different function, so the shapes of the yoga postures have a very different function from those of dance, gymnastics, and acrobatics.

In yoga the shapes of the postures act like a lens bringing the mind into focus. Each posture brings the mind to bear on a different set of muscles, a different pattern of muscular relationships. These muscles are activated by subtle internal adjustments that establish the structural and energetic integrity of the postures. Establishing these adjustments transforms the postures from shapes to postures, from exercise to spiritual practice.

The instructions for each posture are divided into steps. These steps are not simply descriptive divisions. They can also be used as the basis for your step-by-step, breath-synchronized entry into the postures.

THE ENERGIZING POSTURES

The following seven postures constitute the core of the **Energizing Practice**. The remaining posture of the **Energizing Practice, The Big Chill (R6)**, is to be found in the **Rejuvenating Postures** section.

E1 Standing Pose

This posture is good for centering
the mind in the body. Use the flow
of the breath to bring your mind
into a deep awareness of the body.
The pose awakens the feet, legs,
arms, and hands.

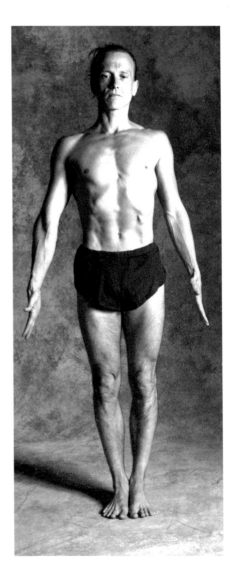

1. Stand upright at the front of your mat with your feet together.
2. Spread your body weight evenly across your feet so that you have the same amount of weight on your heels as on the balls of your feet, on the inner edges of your feet as on the outer edges, and on your left foot as on your right. Broaden the balls of your feet and heels, and lift the arches of your feet.
3. To fully ground your feet and straighten your legs, suck your thigh muscles into the bone so that the backs of your knees open and your kneecaps lift.
4. Soften your buttocks, your pelvic floor, and your groins and lift your hipbones, while drawing your anus and sacrum in by flattening your pubic abdomen. Soften the core of your body, keeping your eyes, ears, and anus passive.
5. Broaden your ribcrests and suck your solar plexus in; lift your ribcage away from your pelvis, lengthening your spine and abdomen, and raise your armpits while relaxing your shoulders.
6. Extend your neck straight up out of your shoulder girdle.
7. Lengthen your arms downwards out of your armpits, broadening your palms and lengthening your fingers.
8. Broaden your collarbones and open your chest.
9. Look straight in front of you.

Hold with the core of your body soft, your solar plexus and anus drawn in, spine and waist long, chest open, and eyes, ears, and anus passive. Keep your legs strong, the balls of your feet and heels broad, and arches lifting. Feel your breath while being aware of the dynamic of your whole body. Hold until ready to release.

E2 Mountain Pose

This posture opens the lungs and lengthens the spine and abdomen easily and effortlessly through the action of the arms. Keep the shoulders relaxed and away from the ears. It awakens the feet, legs, arms, and hands.

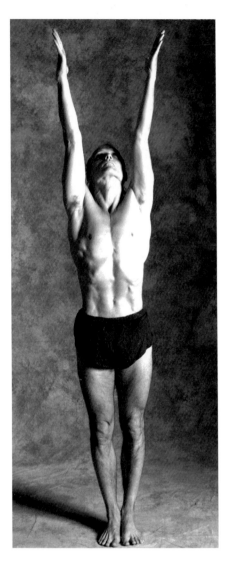

94

1. Stand upright at the front of your mat with your feet together.
2. Spread your body weight evenly across your feet so that you have the same amount of weight on your heels as on the balls of your feet, on the inner edges of your feet as on the outer edges, and on your left foot as on your right. Broaden the balls of your feet and your heels, and lift the arches of your feet.
3. To fully ground your feet and straighten your legs, suck your thigh muscles into the bone so that the backs of your knees open and your kneecaps lift.
4. Soften your buttocks, your pelvic floor, and your groins and lift your hipbones, while drawing your anus and sacrum in by flattening your pubic abdomen. Soften the core of your body, keeping your eyes, ears, and anus passive.
5. Broaden your ribcrests and suck your solar plexus in; lift your ribcage away from your pelvis, lengthening your spine and abdomen, and raise your armpits while relaxing your shoulders.
6. Extend your neck straight up out of your shoulder girdle, and roll your shoulders back and down.
7. Lengthen your arms alongside your ears, broadening your palms and lengthening your fingers.
8. Broaden your collarbones and open your chest.
9. Look up along your fingers.

Hold with the core of your body soft, solar plexus and anus drawn in, spine and waist long, chest open, and eyes, ears, and anus passive. Keep your legs strong, the balls of your feet and heels broad, and arches lifting. Feel your breath while being aware of the dynamic of your whole body. Hold until ready to release.

E3 Chair Pose

This posture develops heat, strengthens the thighs, and develops the feet. Keep the shoulders relaxed and away from the ears.

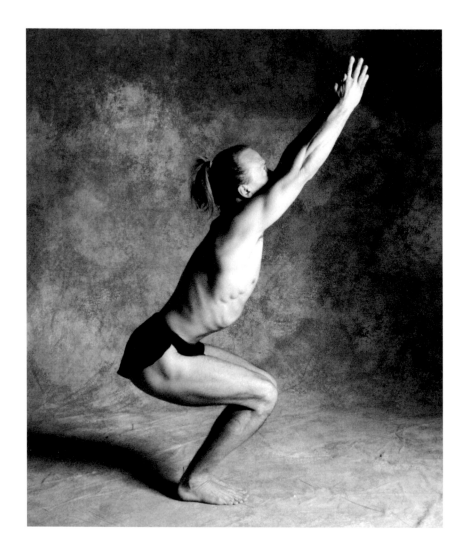

1. Stand upright at the front of your mat with your feet together.
2. Spread your body weight evenly across your feet so that you have the same amount of weight on your heels as on the balls of your feet, on the inner edges of your feet as on the outer edges, and on your left foot as on your right. Broaden the balls of your feet and your heels, and lift the arches of your feet.
3. Pressing your inner ankle bones and inner knees together to activate your inner thighs, bend your legs until your thighs are as close to parallel to the floor as possible.
4. Soften your pelvic floor and your groins and lift your hipbones, while drawing your anus and sacrum in by flattening your pubic abdomen. Soften the core of your body, keeping your eyes, ears, and anus passive.
5. Broaden your ribcrests and suck your solar plexus in; lift your ribcage away from your pelvis; raise your arms alongside your ears, pressing your palms together and broadening and lengthening your fingers, while relaxing your shoulders.
6. Broaden your collarbones and open your chest.
7. Look up along your fingers.

Hold with the core of your body soft, solar plexus and anus drawn in, spine and waist long, chest open, and eyes, ears, and anus passive. Keep your legs strong, the balls of your feet and heels broad, and arches lifting. Feel your breath while being aware of the dynamic of your whole body. Hold until ready to release.

E4 Standing Fold

This posture develops the feet and legs, releases the pelvis, and frees the back. Keep the neck fully relaxed without shaking your head. Do not lift straight back up with straight legs. This posture can also be done in exactly the same manner with the feet hip-width apart. Do not pull yourself into your legs, keep pivoting the pelvis, charging the legs, and lengthening the spine.

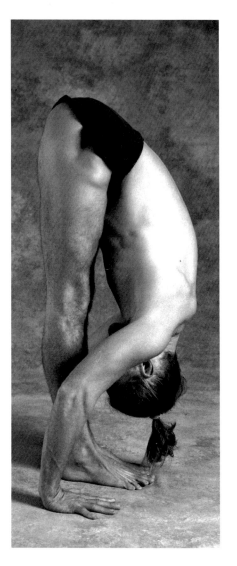

1. Stand upright at the front of your mat with your feet together.
2. Spread your body weight evenly across your feet so that you have the same amount of weight on your heels as on the balls of your feet, on the inner edges of your feet as on the outer edges, and on your left foot as on your right. Broaden the balls of your feet and your heels, and lift the arches of your feet.
3. To fully ground your feet and straighten your legs, suck your thigh muscles into the bone so that the backs of your knees open and your kneecaps lift.
4. Soften your buttocks, pelvic floor, and groins and lift your hipbones while drawing your anus and sacrum in by flattening your pubic abdomen. Soften the core of your body, keeping your eyes, ears, and anus passive.
5. Broaden your ribcrests and suck your solar plexus in; lift your ribcage away from your pelvis, lengthening your spine and abdomen, and raise your armpits while relaxing your shoulders.
6. Keeping your legs straight and strong, pivot your pelvis so your ribs come close to your thighs, keeping your spine and abdomen long and passive.
7. Take your hands to the floor, or hold your shins or ankles, and lengthen your upper arms to draw your trunk further toward your feet. Do not force your ribs into your legs.
8. Relax your shoulders, neck, and back, keeping your legs strong and straight, and your feet alive and active.

Hold with the core of your body soft, solar plexus and anus drawn in, spine and waist long, chest open, and eyes, ears, and anus passive. Keep your legs strong, the balls of your feet and heels broad, and arches lifting. Feel your breath while being aware of the dynamic of your whole body. Hold until ready to release.

Release through **Chair Pose (E3)** without holding.

E5 Leg Raises

This posture develops the back, abdominal, and thigh muscles. Keep the face, neck, shoulders, and lower back relaxed.

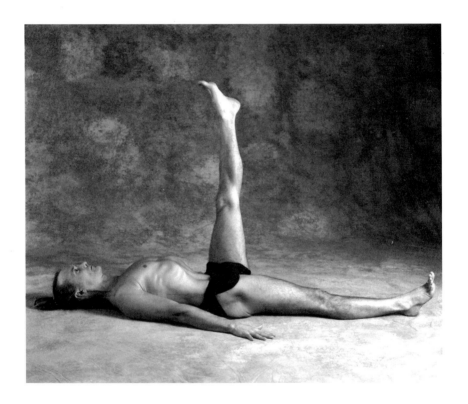

1. Lie flat on your back with your body symmetrical and relaxed, shoulders away from your ears, lower back soft and dropping, but not forced, toward the floor.
2. Extend your arms alongside your trunk and press your palms into the floor, lengthening your fingers. Soften the core of your body, keeping your eyes, ears, and anus passive.
3. Lengthen your abdomen, broaden your ribcrests, and suck your solar plexus in as you take your ribcage away from the pelvis while drawing your anus and sacrum in by flattening your pubic abdomen.
4. Activate your legs by sucking the muscles into the bone, lengthening the front of your ankle and your inner heel while broadening the ball of your foot.
5. As you exhale raise one leg slowly up until it reaches its highest point, keeping both legs straight and strong, your core soft.
6. As you inhale lower the leg slowly until it reaches the floor, keeping both legs straight and strong, and your core soft.

101

Change legs and repeat, alternating your legs in time with your breath while being aware of the dynamic of your whole body, keeping the core of your body soft, and your ears, eyes, and anus passive.

E6 The Bridge

This posture is a back bend. Be sure to use your foundation well and keep your lower back soft. The foundation is the feet, hands, shoulders, and neck.

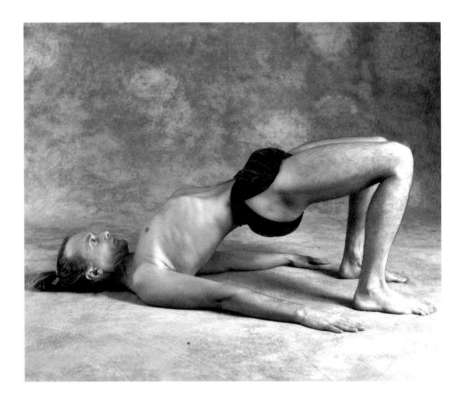

1. Lie flat on your back with your body symmetrical and relaxed, shoulders away from your ears, and your lower back soft and dropping toward the floor.
2. Extend your arms alongside your trunk and press your palms into the floor, lengthening your fingers.
3. Bend your legs and bring your feet in against your buttock bones, knees up and apart above your feet.
4. Activate your feet by pressing the balls of your big and little toes and your inner and outer heels strongly into the floor, so that the balls of your feet and heels broaden and the arches of your feet lift.
5. Lengthen your abdomen, broaden your ribcrests, and suck your solar plexus in as you take your ribcage away from your pelvis; draw your anus and sacrum in by flattening your pubic abdomen and soften the core of your body, keeping your eyes, ears, and anus passive.
6. As you inhale, slowly raise your pelvis and then your spine as high off the floor as you can, while pressing firmly down with your hands and feet.
7. As you exhale lower yourself back down, vertebra by vertebra, buttocks last, keeping your feet in and knees up.
8. Repeat until you have established your maximum movement and then hold your trunk up while breathing slowly, being aware of the dynamic of your whole body, with the feet and hands alive and pressing down, your core soft, and eyes, ears, and anus passive.

Release slowly to the floor on an exhalation, vertebra by vertebra, buttocks last, keeping your feet in and knees up; extend the legs one after the other.

E7 Lying Twist

This posture softens the back and is a counterpose to and preparation for backbends. Keep the straight arm long to ground the top of your body, otherwise the movement of the knee will not bring a full rotation of the spine.

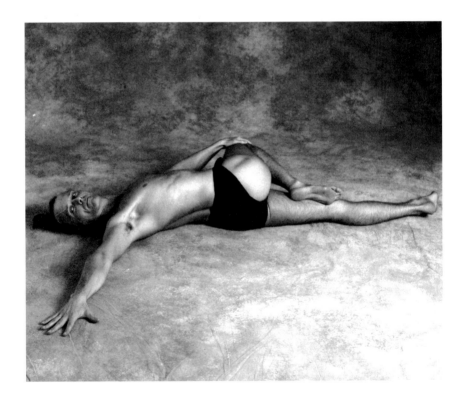

1. Lie flat on your back with your body symmetrical and relaxed, shoulders away from your ears, lower back soft and dropping toward the floor.
2. Extend your arms out at right angles from your trunk, pressing your palms into the floor to keep your arms long and active.
3. Bend your right leg and place your foot flat on the floor, so that it touches the inside of your left knee.
4. Raise your left hip slightly off the floor and, tucking it back and under, take your right knee across the line of your body toward the floor to your left.
5. Place your left hand on the right knee and very gently press it towards the floor; simultaneously extend your right arm out of the armpit, pressing the right shoulder down into the floor.
6. Look along your right arm.

Hold with the core of your body soft, and your eyes, ears, and anus passive as you feel your breath. After a while, release and repeat on the other side.

THE ENERGIZING PRACTICE

This practice will wake you up, charge you up and soften your body. Great for first thing in the morning or any time you need a boost of energy. Best not to do it late at night unless you are going out partying.

E1   E2

Alternate between these two on the breath.

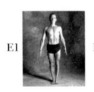

E1   E3

Alternate between the two on the breath.

 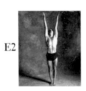

E1   E2   E4   E3   E1

Flow from one to the next on the breath, then repeat.

E3

E5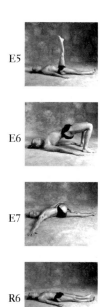

E6

E7

R6

Postures

THE GROUNDING POSTURES

These six postures constitute the core of the **Grounding Practice**. The opening postures of the **Grounding Practice** are to be found in the **Energizing Postures** section. The closing postures of the **Grounding Practice** are to be found in the **Rejuvenating Postures** section.

G1 Triangle Pose

This simple posture awakens the whole body while grounding you. Try to feel the connections between each part of the body.

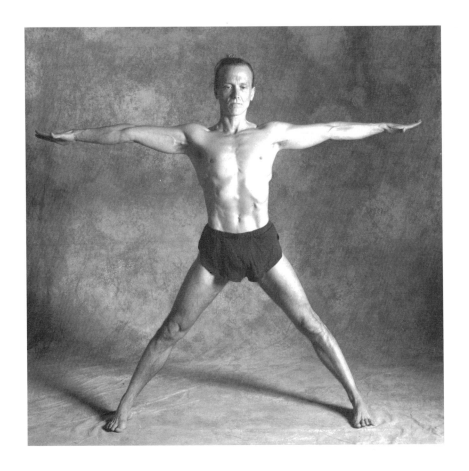

1. Stand with your feet wide apart and parallel to each other.
2. Spread your body weight evenly across your feet so that you have the same amount of weight on your heels as on the balls of your feet, on the inner edges of your feet as on the outer edges, and on your left foot as on your right. Broaden the balls of your feet and your heels, and lift the arches of your feet.
3. To fully ground your feet and straighten your legs, suck your thigh muscles into the bone so that the backs of your knees open and your kneecaps lift and hit the inner bones of the knees away from each other while lifting the inner ankles.
4. Soften your buttocks, your pelvic floor, and your groins and lift your hipbones, while drawing your anus and sacrum in by flattening your pubic abdomen. Soften the core of your body, keeping your eyes, ears, and anus passive.
5. Broaden your ribcrests and suck your solar plexus in; lift your ribcage away from your pelvis, lengthening your spine and abdomen, and raise your armpits while relaxing your shoulders.
6. Extend your neck straight up out of your shoulder girdle.
7. Extend your arms parallel to the floor, broadening your palms and lengthening your fingers.
8. Broaden your collarbones and open your chest.
9. Look straight in front of you.

Hold with the core of your body soft, solar plexus, and anus drawn in, your spine and waist long, chest open, and eyes, ears, and anus passive. Keep your legs strong, the balls of your feet and heels broad, and arches lifting. Feel your breath while being aware of the dynamic of your whole body. Hold until ready to release back to **Standing Pose (E1).**

G2 Gazing Pose

This posture is an extension of **Triangle Pose**. It teaches the feet and legs how to support and lengthen the spine.

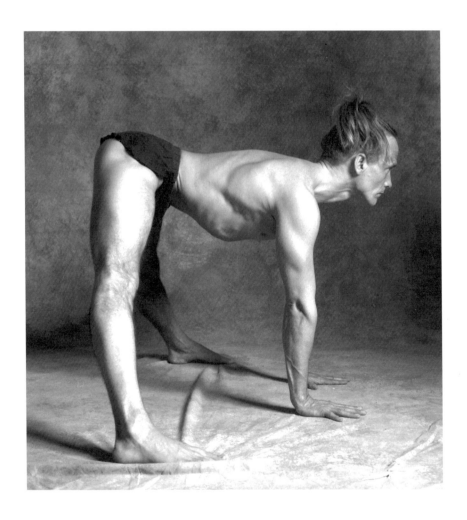

1. Stand with your feet wide apart and parallel to each other.
2. Spread your body weight evenly across your feet so that you have the same amount of weight on your heels as on the balls of your feet, on the inner edges of your feet as on the outer edges, and on your left foot as on your right. Broaden the balls of your feet and your heels, and lift the arches of your feet.
3. To fully ground your feet and straighten your legs, suck your thigh muscles into the bone so that the backs of your knees open and your kneecaps lift and hit the inner bones of the knees away from each other while lifting the inner ankles.
4. Soften your buttocks, your pelvic floor and your groins, and lift your hipbones while drawing your anus and sacrum in by flattening your pubic abdomen. Soften the core of your body, keeping your eyes, ears, and anus passive.
5. Broaden your ribcrests and suck your solar plexus in; lift your ribcage away from your pelvis, lengthening your spine and abdomen, and raise your armpits while relaxing your shoulders.
6. Extend your neck straight up out of your shoulder girdle and your arms parallel to the floor, broadening your palms and lengthening your fingers, while broadening your collarbones.
7. Keeping your legs strong, pivot your pelvis and take your hands to the floor.
8. Lifting your buttock bones to lengthen your legs, roll your pubic bone toward your anus, lengthen your waist and spine out of your pelvis, and lift your armpits.
9. Raise your head, look forward, and open your chest.

Hold with the core of your body soft, solar plexus and anus drawn in, and your eyes, ears, and anus passive. Feel your breathing, while being aware of the dynamic of your whole body. Hold until ready to release back to **Triangle Pose (G1)**.

G3 Leg Stretch

This posture is an extension of **Gazing Pose**. It relaxes the back and spine while developing the legs and feet. Keep the legs strong, feet alive, and your back, shoulders, and neck relaxed.

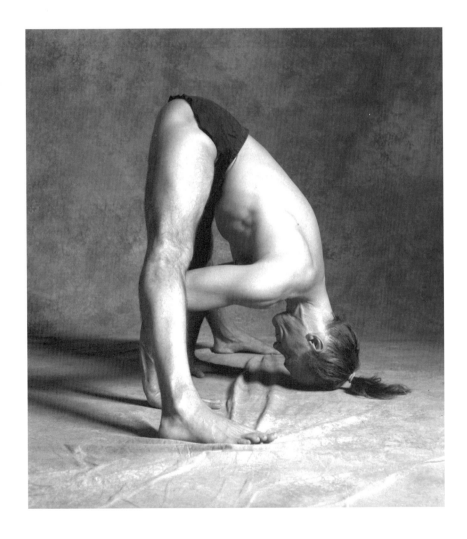

1. Stand with your feet wide apart and parallel to each other.
2. Spread your body weight evenly across your feet so that you have the same amount of weight on your heels as on the balls of your feet, on the inner edges of your feet as on the outer edges, and on your left foot as on your right. Broaden the balls of your feet and your heels, and lift the arches of your feet.
3. To fully ground your feet and straighten your legs, suck your thigh muscles into the bone, so that the backs of your knees open and your kneecaps lift and hit the inner bones of the knees away from each other, while lifting the inner ankles.
4. Soften your buttocks, your pelvic floor, and your groins and lift your hipbones, while drawing your anus and sacrum in by flattening your pubic abdomen. Soften the core of your body, keeping your eyes, ears, and anus passive.
5. Broaden your ribcrests and suck your solar plexus in; lift your ribcage away from your pelvis, lengthening your spine and abdomen, and raise your armpits while relaxing your shoulders.
6. Extend your neck straight up out of your shoulder girdle and your arms parallel to the floor, broadening your palms and lengthening your fingers, while broadening your collarbones.
7. With your legs strong, pivot your pelvis and take your hands to the floor.
8. Lifting your buttock bones to lengthen your legs, roll your pubic bone toward your anus and lengthen your waist and spine out of your pelvis; lift your armpits.
9. Lower your head to the floor between your hands and broaden the ribcrests, while lengthening the waist and spine, and relaxing your shoulders, spine, and lower back.

Hold with the core of your body soft, solar plexus and anus drawn in, and eyes, ears, and anus passive. Feel your breathing, aware of the dynamic of your whole body. Hold until ready to release back to **Triangle Pose (G1)**.

G4 Supported Lunge

This posture aligns the pelvis through the work of the feet and legs. Work from the feet, through the legs to the spine, via the pelvis. Keep the front knee centered over the ankle bone.

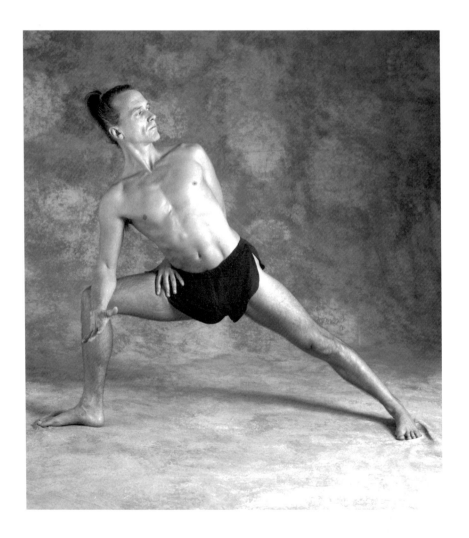

1. Stand with your feet wide apart and parallel to each other.
2. Turn your right foot 90 degrees on its heel, while turning the left foot in about 15 degrees, and line up the right heel with the left ankle. Spread your body weight evenly across your feet as you engage them by broadening the balls of your feet.
3. Rolling your left hip back away from your front leg, ground your feet by sucking your thigh muscles in so that the four corners of your feet are pressing down and the backs of your knees open and your kneecaps lift.
4. Soften your buttocks, pelvic floor and groins, and lift your hipbones while drawing your anus and sacrum in by flattening your pubic abdomen. Soften the core of your body, keeping your eyes, ears, and anus passive.
5. Broaden your ribcrests and suck your solar plexus in; lift your ribcage away from your pelvis, lengthening your spine and abdomen, and extend your arms parallel to the floor, palms broad, fingers long, looking along the right arm while broadening your collarbones.
6. Keeping the left leg straight by rolling the outer edge of the knee back, bend the right leg until you have a right angle — thighbone parallel to the floor, shinbone perpendicular, knee directly above the ankle. Adjust your feet spacing if you need to.
7. Without changing your legs or pelvis, extend your right arm forward, lengthening your waist until the armpit is above the knee.
8. Taking your left arm behind your waist, bend your right arm and place your elbow on your right thigh by the knee. Lengthen the right side of your body from the hip to the armpit, keeping the shoulder relaxed.
9. Turn and look over your left shoulder as you turn the whole of the left side of your body away from the floor, from the shinbone to the armpit.

Hold with the core of your body soft, solar plexus and anus drawn in, and eyes, ears, and anus passive. Feel your breathing while being aware of the dynamic of your whole body. Hold until ready to release back to **Triangle Pose (G1)**. Repeat on the left.

Postures

G5 Revolving Lunge

This posture gives a simple, satisfying twist to the spine, while developing the feet and legs and freeing the pelvis. Work from the feet, through the legs to the spine, via the pelvis. Keep the front knee centered over the ankle bone.

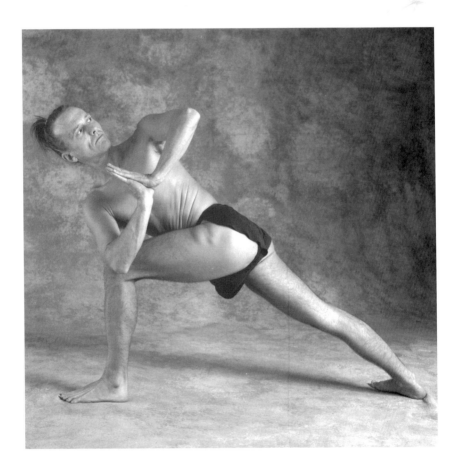

1. Stand with your feet wide apart and parallel to each other, hands on hips.
2. Turn your right foot 90 degrees on its heel, while turning the left foot in 45–75 degrees so that the heel turns a long way back; line up the right heel with the left ankle. Spread your body weight evenly across your feet, engaging them by broadening the balls of your feet.
3. Turn your trunk forward, bringing your left hip in line with your right, and ground your feet by sucking your thigh muscles in so that the four corners of your feet are pressing down and the backs of your knees open and the kneecaps lift.
4. Soften your buttocks, pelvic floor, and groins, and lift your hipbones while drawing your anus and sacrum in by flattening your pubic abdomen. Soften the body core, keeping eyes, ears, and anus passive.
5. Broaden your ribcrests and suck your solar plexus in; lift your ribcage away from your pelvis, lengthening your spine and abdomen.
6. Keeping the left leg straight by rolling the inner edge of the knee back, bend the right leg until you have a right angle—thighbone parallel to the floor, shinbone perpendicular, knee directly above the ankle. Adjust your feet spacing if you need to. Keep your pelvis turning.
7. Without changing your legs or pelvis, extend your left arm forward and rotate your spine, lengthening your waist until your armpit is above the knee.
8. Place the point of your left elbow on the outside of your right knee, and press the right palm onto the left with your forearms in a straight line.
9. Turn and look over your right shoulder, turning your right armpit toward the ceiling while lengthening your waist and spine, and turning your left groin back with the leg straight and inner edge of the knee hitting back.

Hold with the core of your body soft, solar plexus and anus drawn in, and eyes, ears, and anus passive. Feel your breathing while being aware of the dynamic of your whole body. Hold until ready to release back to **Triangle Pose (G1)**. Repeat on the left.

Postures

G6 Warrior

This posture awakens the whole body while developing the legs and opening the pelvis and groins. Work from the feet, through the legs to the spine, via the pelvis. Keep the armpits directly above their respective hipbones. Keep the front knee centered over the ankle bone.

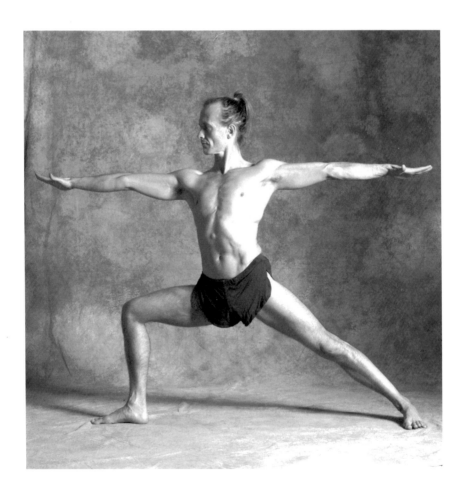

1. Stand with your feet wide apart and parallel to each other.
2. Turn your right foot 90 degrees on its heel, while turning the left foot in about 15 degrees, and line up the right heel with the left ankle. Spread your body weight evenly across your feet and broaden the balls of your feet and your heels; lift the arches of your feet.
3. Rolling your left hip back away from your front leg, ground your feet by sucking your thigh muscles in so that the four corners of your feet are pressing down and the backs of your knees open and the kneecaps lift.
4. Soften your buttocks, pelvic floor, and your groins, and lift your hipbones while drawing your anus and sacrum in by flattening your pubic abdomen. Soften the core of your body, keeping your eyes, ears, and anus passive.
5. Broaden your ribcrests and suck your solar plexus in; lift your ribcage away from your pelvis, lengthening your spine and abdomen, and extend your arms parallel to the floor, palms broad, fingers long, looking along the right arm while broadening your collarbones.
6. Keeping the left leg straight by rolling the outer edge of the knee back, bend the right leg until you have a right angle—thighbone parallel to the floor, shinbone perpendicular, knee directly above the ankle. Adjust your feet spacing if you need to.
7. Look along your right arm.

Hold with the core of your body soft, solar plexus and anus drawn in, and eyes, ears, and anus passive. Feel your breathing while being aware of the dynamic of your whole body. Hold until ready to release back to **Triangle Pose (G1)**. Repeat on the left.

THE GROUNDING PRACTICE

This practice should be your core practice. Best done in the morning, it can also be done later in the day, but better not late at night.

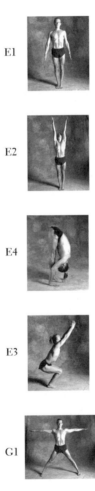

E1

E2

E4

E3

G1

G2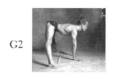

G3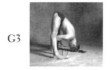

G4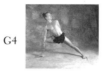

G5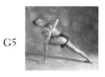

G6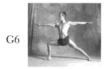

E7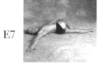

R1

R2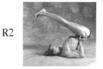

Postures

THE OPENING POSTURES

These 13 postures constitute the **Opening Practice**. This is completed with the **Easy Pose** and **The Big Chill** from the **Rejuvenating Postures**.

01 The Staff

This posture warms up the spine, opens the pelvis, energizes the trunk, and awakens the whole body. The foundation is the backs of the legs and heels, the hands, and the buttock bones.

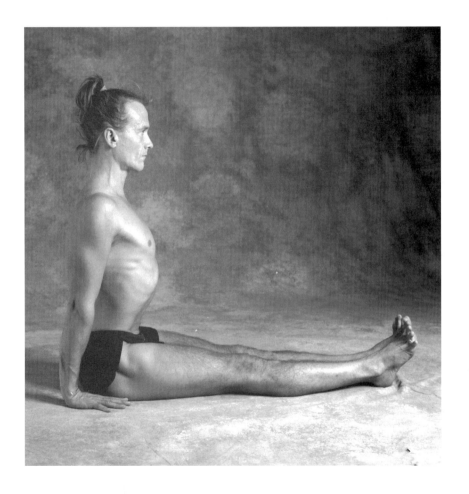

1. Sit on the floor with your legs relaxed and stretched out in front of you.
2. Spread the flesh of your buttocks so that your buttock bones are both clearly on the floor.
3. Place your palms on the floor by your buttocks with your fingers pointing toward your feet.
4. Bring your inner heels, the balls of your big toes, and your inner ankles together.
5. Broaden the balls of your feet from the center and lightly extend your toes upward as you lengthen your front ankle and inner heel.
6. Suck your thigh muscles into the bones so that the backs of your knees open and your thigh and shinbones go down.
7. Pressing with your palms, come to the front edge of your buttock bones and, flattening your pubic abdomen with your anus soft, broaden your ribcrests as you suck your solar plexus in; lift and open your chest, lengthening your waist and spine.
8. Lifting your armpits roll your shoulders away from your ears, and your shoulderblades down your back.
9. Look at your big toes.

Hold while following the flow of your breath, your spine long, chest open, the core of your body soft, and a strong charge in your feet, legs, arms, and trunk. Release when ready.

02 Raised Leg Pose

This posture warms up the spine, leg, and pelvis. The foundation is the relaxed foot and shin, the hand, and the buttock bones.

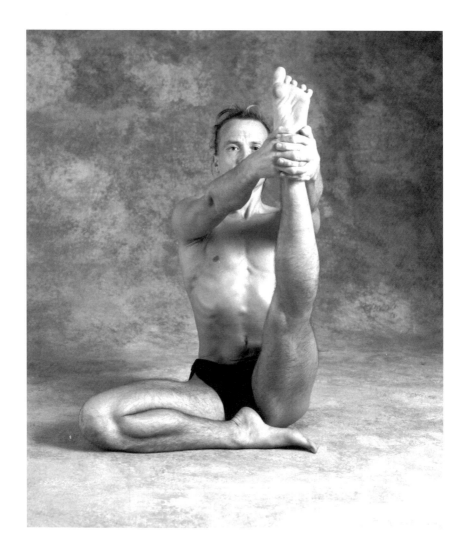

1. Sit on the floor with your legs stretched out in front of you.
2. Bend your right leg and place your heel by the left buttock bone.
3. Bend your left leg and catch hold of the heel in both hands.
4. Straighten your left leg, sucking the thigh muscles in, lengthening the front ankle and inner heel, broadening the ball of the foot, and extending your toes.
5. Coming to the front edge of your buttock bone, flatten the pubic abdomen, keeping your anus soft; broaden your ribcrests as you suck your solar plexus in, lift your ribcage and open your chest, lengthening your waist and spine.
6. Lift your armpits, roll your shoulders away from your ears, and your shoulderblades down your back; straighten your arms.
7. Use the triangular dynamic between your leg, arms, and trunk to continuously lengthen your spine.
8. Look at your foot.

Hold while following the flow of your breath; your spine long, chest open, the core of your body soft, and a strong charge in your raised leg and foot, arms, and trunk. Release when ready, then repeat on the other side.

03 Side Raised Leg Pose

This posture warms up the spine, leg, and pelvis. The foundation is the relaxed foot and shin, the hand, and the buttock bones.

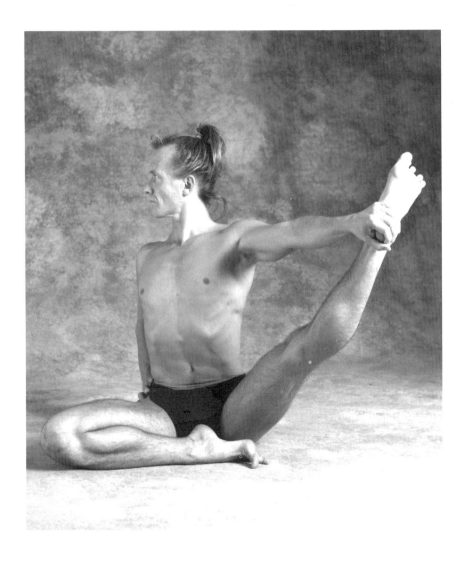

1. Sit on the floor with your legs stretched out in front of you.
2. Bend your right leg and place your heel by the left buttock bone.
3. Bend your left leg and catch your inner heel in your left hand, placing your right hand by your right buttock.
4. Straighten your left leg, sucking the thigh muscles in, lengthening the front ankle and inner heel, broadening the ball of the foot, and extending your toes.
5. Coming to the front edge of your buttock bone, flatten the pubic abdomen, keeping your anus soft; broaden your ribcrests as you suck your solar plexus in, lift your ribcage and open your chest, lengthening your waist and spine.
6. Lift your armpits, roll your shoulders away from your ears, and your shoulderblades down your back; straighten your arms.
7. Turning your head to the right, take your left leg out to the left, keeping it centered in the hip socket as much as possible.
8. Use the triangular dynamic between your leg, arm, and trunk to continuously lengthen your spine.
9. Look over your right shoulder.

Hold while following the flow of your breath, with your spine long, chest open, the core of your body soft, and a strong charge in your raised leg and foot, arms, and trunk. Release when ready, then repeat on the other side.

04 Raised Leg Twist

This posture warms up the spine, leg, and pelvis. The foundation is the relaxed foot and shin, the hand, and the buttock bones.

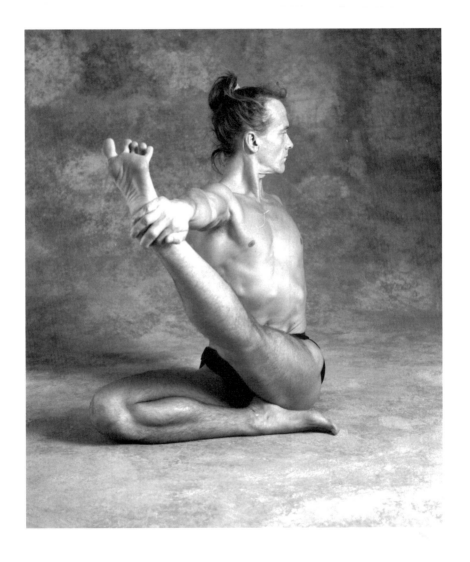

1. Sit on the floor with your legs stretched out in front of you.
2. Bend your right leg and place your heel by the left buttock bone.
3. Bend your left leg and catch the outer heel in your right hand, placing your left hand by your left buttock.
4. Straighten your left leg, sucking the thigh muscles in, lengthening the front ankle and inner heel, broadening the ball of the foot, and extending your toes.
5. Coming to the front edge of your buttock bone, flatten the pubic abdomen keeping your anus soft; broaden your ribcrests as you suck your solar plexus in, lift your ribcage, and open your chest, lengthening your waist and spine.
6. Lift your armpits, roll your shoulders away from your ears, and your shoulderblades down your back; straighten your arms.
7. Turning your head to the left, take your left leg across the line of your body to the right.
8. Use the triangular dynamic between your leg, arm, and trunk to continuously lengthen your spine.
9. Look over your left shoulder.

Hold while following the flow of your breath, your spine long, chest open, the core of your body soft, and a strong charge in your raised leg and foot, arms, and trunk. Release when ready, then repeat on the other side.

05 Boat Pose

This posture lengthens and develops the back, abdomen, and legs. To make it easier in the beginning you can bend the leg until the shin is parallel to the floor. Or you can support the leg with the arms through the back of the knee. The foundation is the relaxed foot and shin, and the buttock bones.

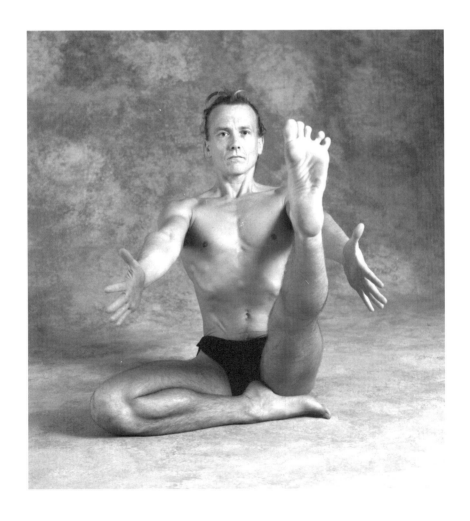

1. Sit on the floor with your legs stretched out in front of you.
2. Bend your right leg and place your heel by the left buttock bone.
3. Bend your left leg and catch the heel in both hands.
4. Straighten your left leg, sucking the thigh muscles in, lengthening the front ankle and inner heel, broadening the ball of the foot, and extending your toes.
5. Coming to the front edge of your buttock bone, flatten the pubic abdomen keeping your anus soft; broaden your ribcrests as you suck your solar plexus in, lift your ribcage, and open your chest, lengthening your waist and spine.
6. Lift your armpits, roll your shoulders away from your ears, and your shoulderblades down your back; straighten your arms.
7. Use the triangular dynamic between your leg, arms, and trunk to continuously lengthen your spine.
8. Let go of your foot and extend your arms parallel to the floor, keeping your leg strong and in the air.
9. Look at your foot.

Hold while following the flow of your breath, your spine long, chest open, the core of your body soft, and a strong charge in your raised leg and foot, arms, and trunk. Release when ready, then repeat on the other side.

06 Easy Twist

This posture softens the spine and back muscles. Do not force the spine into the twist. Move freely with the breath, emphasizing the elongation of the spine. The foundation is the relaxed bent leg, the up-leg foot, and the buttock bones.

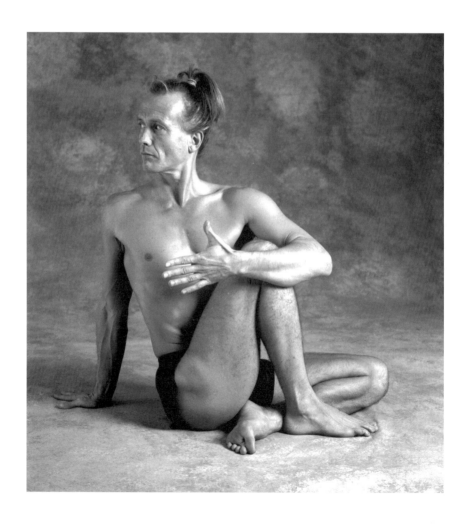

1. Sit on the floor with your legs stretched out in front of you.
2. Bend your left leg and place your heel by the right buttock bone with your left knee on the floor.
3. Bend your right leg and place the heel against the left ankle bone, with your right knee up in front of you.
4. Wrap your left arm deeply round your right knee or shin.
5. Take your right hand back and round behind you and place the palm on the floor behind your sacrum.
6. With both buttock bones on the floor, press your right foot into the floor.
7. Flattening your pubic abdomen, suck your anus in and, broadening your ribcrests, suck your solar plexus in as you lift your ribcage and open your chest.
8. Lift into your armpits, roll your shoulders away from your ears, and your shoulderblades down your back.
9. Look over your right shoulder.

Hold while following the flow of your breath, your spine long, chest open, the core of your body soft, and a strong charge in your arms and trunk. Release when ready, then repeat on the other side.

07 Twist

This posture softens the spine and back muscles, and opens the pelvis. Do not force the spine into the twist. Move freely with the breath, emphasizing the elongation of the spine. The foundation is the straight leg and heel, the bent leg foot, and the buttock bones.

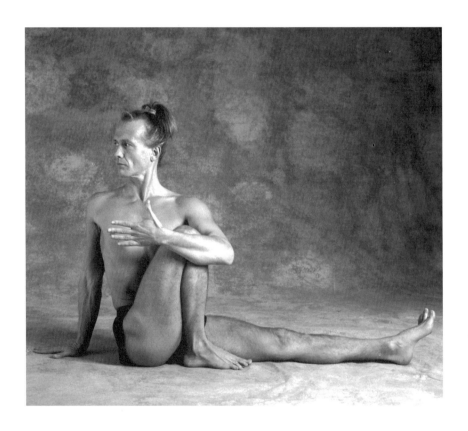

1. Sit on the floor with your legs stretched out in front of you.
2. Bend your right leg and place the heel against the right buttock bone, with your right knee up in front of you.
3. Center your left foot on the heel, lengthen the front ankle and the inner heel, broaden the ball of the foot, and suck the thigh muscles into the bone so that the back of the knee opens and the shin and thighbones go down.
4. Wrap your left arm deeply round your right knee or shin.
5. Take your right hand back and round behind you and place the palm on the floor behind your sacrum.
6. With both buttock bones on the floor, press your right foot into the floor.
7. Flattening your pubic abdomen, suck your anus in and, broadening your ribcrests, suck your solar plexus in as you lift your ribcage and open your chest.
8. Lift into your armpits; roll your shoulders away from your ears, and your shoulderblades down your back.
9. Look over your right shoulder.

Hold while following the flow of your breath, your spine long, chest open, the core of your body soft, and a strong charge in your left leg, arms, and trunk. Release when ready, then repeat on the other side.

139

08 One Leg Extension

This posture stretches the hamstrings, releases the pelvis, softens the back, and lengthens the spine. The foundation is the straight leg and heel, and the buttock bone.

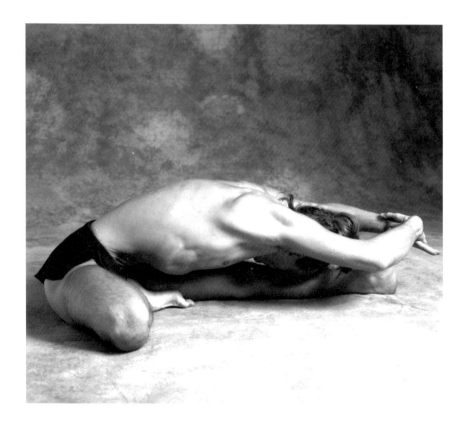

1. Sit on the floor with your legs relaxed and stretched out in front of you.
2. Bend your right leg and place its heel in your left groin, so that the foot runs along the inside of your left leg. Soften the skin of your right knee with your hand.
3. Spread the flesh of your buttocks so that your buttock bones are both clearly on the floor.
4. Place your palms on the floor by your buttocks with your fingers pointing toward your feet.
5. Broaden the ball of your left foot from the center and lightly extend your toes upward, as you lengthen your front ankle and inner heel.
6. Suck your left thigh muscles into the bones so that the back of your knee opens and your thigh and shinbone go down.
7. Pressing with your palms, come to the front edge of your buttock bones and, flattening your pubic abdomen with your anus soft, broaden your ribcrests as you suck your solar plexus in; lift and open your chest, lengthening your waist and spine.
8. Reach forward with both hands and catch your shin, ankle or foot without bending your leg.
9. Gripping with your hands, lift your chest and chin, and lengthen your waist and spine forward and upward as you roll your pubic bone back, keeping your leg strong.
10. Leading with the chin, armpits, and elbows bring your head and trunk forward, allowing them to come quietly down toward your straight leg.
11. Look within.

Hold while following the flow of your breath, your spine long, chest open, the core of your body soft, and a strong charge in the foot, leg, and trunk. Release when ready, and repeat on the other side.

Postures

09 Sitting Splits

This posture opens the groins, frees the pelvis, and develops the legs and feet. The foundation is the backs of the legs and heels, the hands, and the buttock bones.

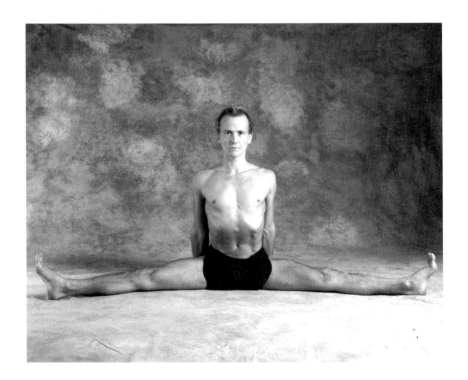

1. Sit on the floor with your legs stretched out to the sides.
2. Place your hands behind your buttocks and, raising them a little off the floor, push your groins forward widening the space between your feet, and stretch and lengthen your legs.
3. With both buttock bones back on the floor, suck your thigh muscles into the bone so that the backs of your knees open and your thighs and shins go down.
4. Broaden the balls of your feet, extend your toes lightly, and lengthen your front ankles and inner heels away from you.
5. Pressing the backs of your legs down and your palms into the floor behind your buttocks, come to the front edge of your buttock bones.
6. Using your arms to lift you, flatten your pubic abdomen with your anus soft; broaden your ribcrests as you suck your solar plexus in, and lift and open your chest, lengthening your waist and spine.
7. Keeping your shoulders relaxed, roll them back and drop your shoulderblades as you lengthen up into your armpits.
8. Look straight ahead.

Hold while following the flow of your breath, your spine long, chest open, the core of your body soft, and a strong charge in the feet, legs, arms, and trunk. Release when ready.

O10 Cobbler

This posture opens the pelvis, groins, and ankles. The foundation is the buttock bones and the legs and feet.

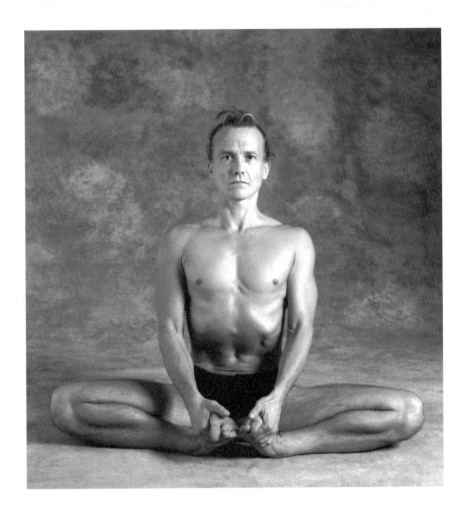

1. Sit on the floor with your legs relaxed in front of you.
2. Bring the soles of your feet together, keeping your knees out to the sides and down by the floor.
3. Place your thumbs on the balls of your big toes, the tips of your fingers on the outer edges of your feet, which should be resting against each other.
4. Pushing up with your fingertips onto the outer bones of your feet, press out with your thumbs on the balls of your big toes, so that your feet open and the knees go down. Do not press your knees down.
5. Using the grip of your hands, lengthen your arms and lift into your armpits, keeping your shoulders relaxed and rolling back; drop your shoulderblades.
6. Flatten your pubic abdomen with your anus soft; broaden your ribcrests as you suck your solar plexus in, and lift and open your chest, lengthening your waist and spine.
7. Keeping your shoulders relaxed roll them back and drop your shoulderblades as you lengthen up into your armpits.
8. Look straight ahead.

145

Hold while following the flow of your breath, your spine long, chest open, the core of your body soft, and a strong charge in the arms and trunk. Release when ready.

011 Balancing Pose

This posture relaxes the brain, develops balance, poise, and the legs and opens the pelvis. The foundation is the buttock bones, *not* the coccyx.

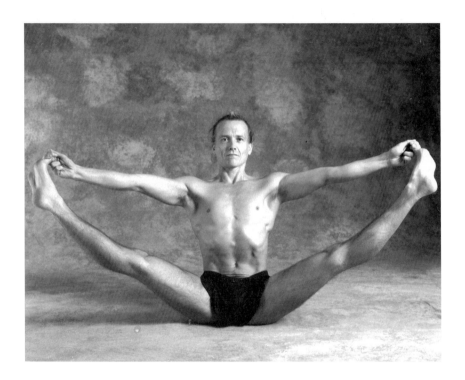

1. Sit on the floor with your legs relaxed in front of you.
2. Bend your legs and take hold of each of your big toes in the thumbs and first two fingers of your hands.
3. Lifting your feet off the floor, balance on your buttocks with your legs still bent.
4. Take your feet away from each other and your trunk, straightening the legs as much as possible.
5. Broaden the balls of your feet, lengthen your toes lightly, and lengthen your front ankles and inner heels away from you. If your legs straighten suck your thigh muscles in so the backs of your knees open.
6. Using the grip of your hands, lengthen your arms and lift into your armpits, keeping your shoulders relaxed and rolling back; drop your shoulderblades.
7. Flatten your pubic abdomen with your anus soft; broaden your ribcrests as you suck your solar plexus in, and lift and open your chest, lengthening your waist and spine.
8. Keeping your shoulders relaxed, roll them back and drop your shoulderblades as you lengthen up into your armpits.
9. Look straight ahead.

Hold while following the flow of your breath, your spine long, chest open, the core of your body soft, and a strong charge in the feet, legs, arms, and trunk. Release when ready.

012 Sitting Fold

This posture stretches the hamstrings, releases the pelvis, softens the back, and lengthens the spine. The foundation is the backs of the legs and heels and the buttock bones. Do not pull yourself into your legs; keep pivoting the pelvis, charging the legs, and lengthening the spine.

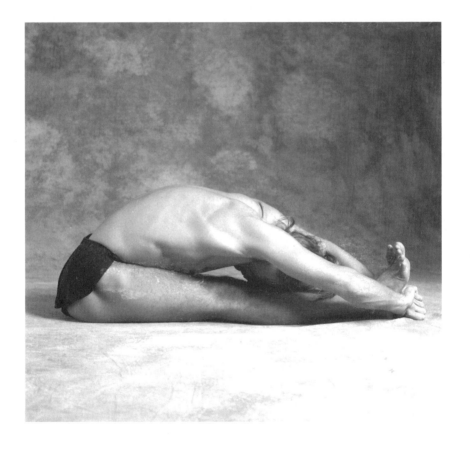

1. Sit on the floor with your legs relaxed and stretched out in front of you.
2. Spread the flesh of your buttocks so that your buttock bones are both clearly on the floor.
3. Place your palms on the floor by your buttcoks with your fingers pointing toward your feet.
4. Bring your inner heels, the balls of your big toes, and your inner ankles together.
5. Broaden the balls of your feet from the center and lightly extend your toes upward, as you lengthen your front ankle and inner heel.
6. Suck your thigh muscles into the bones so that the backs of your knees open and your thigh and shinbones go down.
7. Pressing with your palms, come to the front edge of your buttock bones and, flattening your pubic abdomen with your anus soft, broaden your ribcrests as you suck your solar plexus in; lift and open your chest, lengthening your waist and spine.
8. Reach forward with both hands and catch hold of your shins, ankles or feet without bending your legs.
9. Gripping with your hands, lift your chest and chin, and lengthen your waist and spine forward and upward as you roll your pubic bone back, keeping your legs strong.
10. Leading with the chin, armpits, and elbows, bring your head and trunk forward, allowing them to come quietly down towards your straight legs.
11. Look within.

Hold while following the flow of your breath, your spine long, chest open, the core of your body soft, and a strong charge in the feet, legs, and trunk. Release when ready.

013 Opening Pose

This posture opens the front of the body as a counterposture to the **Sitting Fold**. The foundation is the hands and all of the feet.

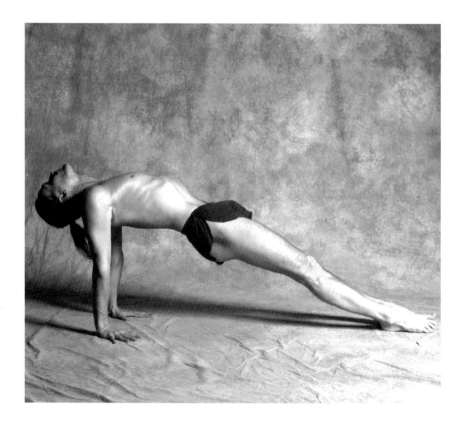

1. Sit on the floor with your legs relaxed and stretched out in front of you.
2. Place your palms on the floor behind your buttocks, with your fingers pointing toward your feet.
3. Bring your inner heels, the balls of your big toes, and your inner ankles together; broaden the balls of your feet from the center and lightly extend your toes upward, as you lengthen your front ankle and inner heel.
4. Suck your thigh muscles into the bones so that the backs of your knees open and your thigh and shinbones go down.
5. Pressing with your palms, straighten your arms and lift your pelvis and spine up from the floor, keeping your legs strong.
6. Stretch the balls of your feet to the floor as you raise your pelvis as high as you can, with your buttocks soft.
7. Lift your chin and, taking your head back, use your hands and arms to lift your top spine and chest.
8. Look within.

Hold with your arms and legs active, core soft, pubic abdomen, and ribcrests broad, following the flow of your breath until ready to release the buttocks back down to the floor.

THE OPENING PRACTICE

This practice can be used when you do not feel very energetic, or when you want to have a more relaxed but deep practice.

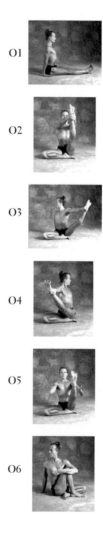

O1

O2

O3

O4

O5

O6

Postures O1–O8 can be done together in a single fluid sequence on one side, and then on the other side in the same way.

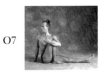

O7

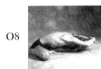

O8

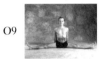

O9

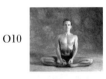

O10

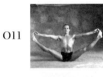

O11

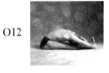

O12

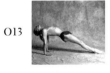

O13

R5

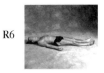

R6

THE REJUVENATING POSTURES

These postures constitute the core of the **Rejuvenating Practice**. However, the opening postures of the **Rejuvenating Practice** are to be found in the **Opening Postures** and the **Energizing Postures** sections.

R1 Embryo Pose

This posture is very relaxing for the whole body. Keep the shoulders away from the ears. Allow the breath to enter the back of the lungs. Take care that there is no pressure in the neck. The foundation is the elbows, the back of the head, and the top of the shoulder girdle.

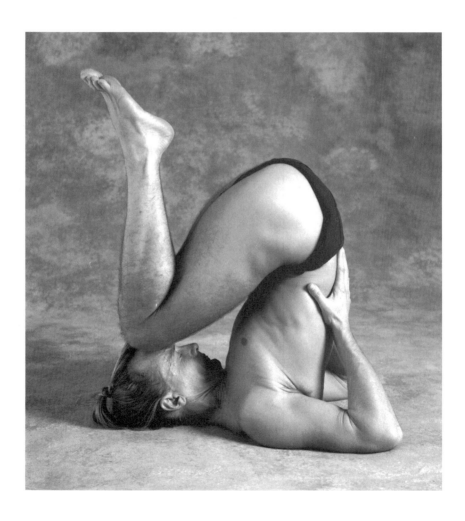

1. Lie on your back, shoulders away from your ears.
2. Stretching your hands away from your body, draw your knees up toward your chest.
3. Pressing down with your hands roll yourself up onto your shoulders, placing your hands on your back.
4. Drop your knees down onto your forehead.
5. Draw your heels in to your buttocks.
6. Look within.

Hold with the whole body relaxed except for the effort required to hold the heels close to the buttocks. Breathe into the back of the lungs, keeping the core of your body soft. When ready to release extend your arms away from you and, with your hands pressing down, roll your spine down from the top to the bottom so that the buttocks land last with legs bent; straighten your legs along the floor, one after the other.

157

R2 Half Shoulderstand

This posture rejuvenates the whole body, lengthens the abdomen, and teaches the shoulders and arms how to lift and support the spine. Keep the shoulders away from the ears. Take care that there is no pressure in the neck. The foundation is the elbows, the back of the head, and the top of the shoulder girdle.

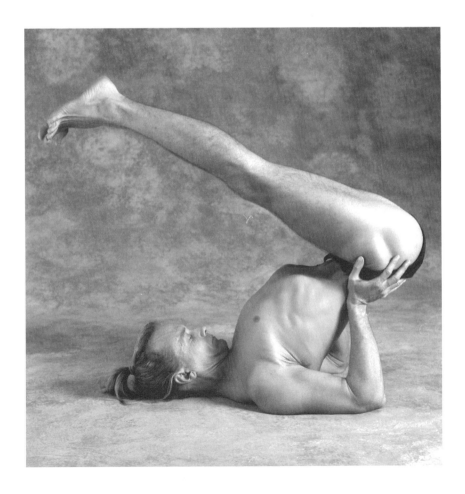

1. Lie on your back, shoulders away from your ears.
2. Stretching your hands away from your body, draw your knees up toward your chest.
3. Pressing down with your hands roll yourself up onto your shoulders, placing your hands on your back.
4. Bend your legs and drop your knees down onto your forehead.
5. Keeping your legs bent, roll your pelvis and legs away from you and slide your hands down your back until they are supporting the rim of your pelvis.
6. With your legs still bent, take your pubic bone as far away from your ribcage as you can, lengthening your waist and gently arching your lower back.
7. Pressing your upper arms and shoulders into the floor, draw the top spine forward and open your chest—broadening across your collarbones, so that your back is now arching in a gentle back bend.
8. Straighten your legs, suck your thigh muscles in, and press your inner ankles together.
9. Look at your ribcrests as you broaden them, while flattening the abdomen.

Hold with the core of your body soft, deepening the hollowness of your abdomen as you broaden your ribcrests and open your chest. When ready to release bend your legs, press your hands to the floor behind you, and roll your spine down from the top to the bottom so the buttocks land last with legs bent; straighten your legs along the floor, one after the other.

R3 Half Plow

This posture relaxes and lengthens the back muscles and rests the legs. Take care that there is no pressure in the neck. Keep the shoulders away from the ears. The foundation is the elbows, the feet, the back of the head, and the top of the shoulder girdle.

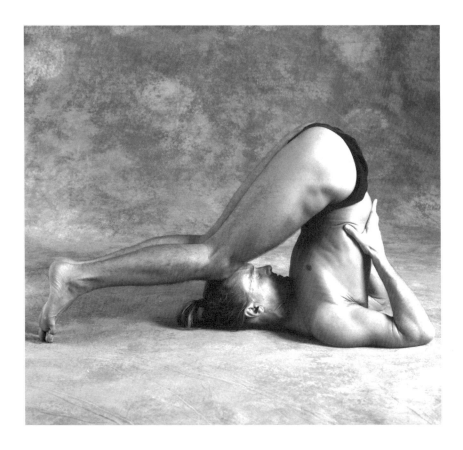

1. Lie on your back, shoulders away from your ears.
2. Stretching your hands away from your body, draw your knees up toward your chest.
3. Pressing down with your hands roll yourself up onto your shoulders, placing your hands on your back.
4. Drop your knees down onto your forehead.
5. Drop your feet toward the floor behind your head, keeping your legs completely relaxed with your knees still on your forehead.
6. Look within.

Hold with the whole body relaxed. Breathe into the back of the lungs, keeping the core of your body soft. When ready to release bend your legs, bringing your heels toward your buttocks, and take your arms the opposite way from your head, hands pressing down; roll your spine down from the top to the bottom so the buttocks land last with legs bent; straighten your legs along the floor, one after the other.

161

R4 Fetus Pose

This posture is very relaxing for the whole body, and gives a deep stretch to the muscles of the back and shoulders. Keep the shoulders away from the ears. Allow the breath to enter the back of the lungs. Take care that there is no pressure in the neck. The whole body should be totally relaxed—no effort anywhere.

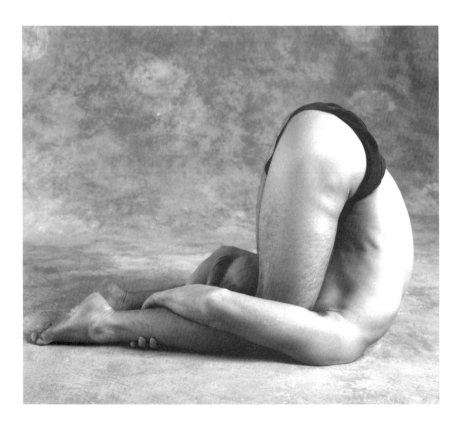

1. Lie on your back, with your shoulders away from your ears.
2. Stretching your hands away from your body, draw your knees up toward your chest.
3. Pressing down with your hands roll yourself up onto your shoulders, placing your hands on your back.
4. Drop your knees down onto your forehead.
5. Drop your feet toward the floor behind your head, keeping your legs completely relaxed with your knees still on your forehead.
6. Stretch your arms back alongside your ears.
7. Drop your knees down onto your arms.
8. If you can, move your arms outside your knees so that your knees come to the ground, then pass each hand over the calf and under the opposite shin.
9. Look within.

Hold with the whole body relaxed. Breathe into the back of the lungs, keeping the core of your body soft. When ready to release bring your heels toward your buttocks, your arms to the other side of your trunk with the hands pressing down, and roll your spine down from the top to the bottom so the buttocks land last with legs bent; straighten your legs along the floor, one after the other.

R5 Easy Pose

This posture is a simple sitting posture in which the body can relax with the mind alert. The foundation is the buttock bones, the ankles, and the shins.

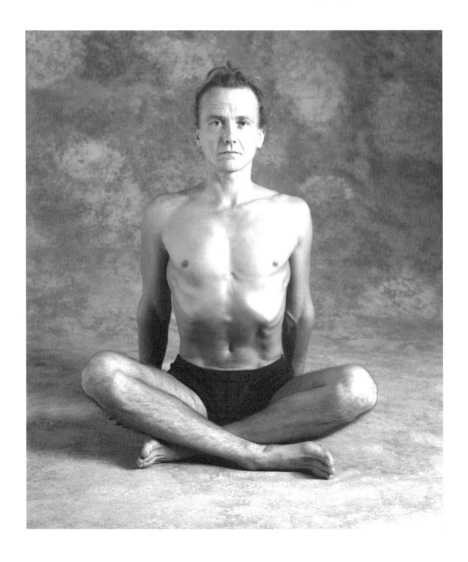

1. Sit on the floor with your legs in front of you.
2. Cross your legs in a relaxed way, so that each foot is resting under and supporting the opposite leg. The legs should not be tightly crossed.
3. Relax your legs, pelvis, abdomen, and face.
4. Place your hands behind your buttocks and use them to roll to the front edge of your buttock bones.
5. Flattening your pubic abdomen, broaden your ribcrests; lift your ribcage and lengthen your waist and spine.
6. Keeping your armpits up, roll your shoulders back and drop your shoulderblades down your back.
7. Look straight ahead, your attention within.

Hold your body still and follow the flow of your breathing, keeping the core of your body soft.

R6 The Big Chill

This posture allows for very deep relaxation, during which gravity can work on lengthening muscle tissue, opening joints, and realigning bones. It also allows the mind to develop the internalization, subtlety, and stability required of meditation.

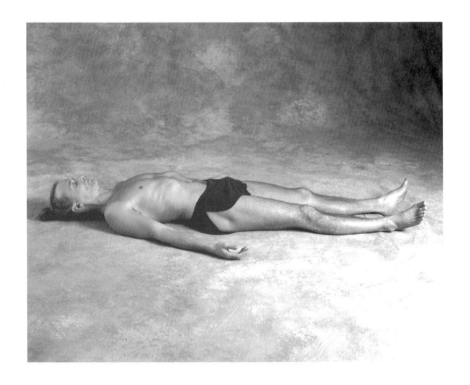

1. Lie symmetrically on your back, arms by your sides.
2. Lift your pelvis and draw your buttocks away from your waist. Soften your lower back as your buttocks come back to the floor.
3. Lengthen your legs out of your pelvis, bringing your heels together. As you relax them, allow the balls of your feet to roll away from each other.
4. Relax your shoulders and draw them away from your ears as you lengthen your neck without constricting the throat.
5. Lengthen your arms out of your armpits alongside you, with your palms up and a little away from your body so that there is space in your armpits.
6. Try to make your body symmetrical by adjusting the left and right sides of you until they feel as much as possible the same.
7. Take your attention deep into your pelvis and gently encourage all the pelvic muscles to relax. As you feel your pelvis softening, with the bones dropping to the floor, focus on releasing your anus and perineum.
8. Take your attention deep into your brain and gently encourage all the cells to soften and relax. Allow your eyes and ears to soften and melt down into your brain, relaxing your jaw and forehead.
9. While continuously encouraging your pelvis and brain to soften more and more, allow their softness to spread effortlessly into the whole of your body.
10. Without any concern for which part of the body is doing what, simply feel your way deeper and deeper into your body so that the presence of your awareness in your body encourages it to relax more and more.

Hold while paying direct attention to all of the sensations inside you as they freely come and go. When ready to release, gently and gradually begin to stretch and flex your fingers and toes, bringing that movement through the wrists and ankles into your arms and legs, shoulders and pelvis, chest and waist, spine and neck. When you have activated all your muscles gently, roll onto your right side until you are ready to sit up.

Postures

THE REJUVENATING PRACTICE

This practice should be done when you are tired, recuperating from illness, or when you are wound up or hyperactive and need to relax and calm down.

O11

O12

O13

E6

E7

R1

R2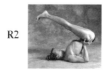

R3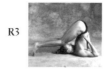

R4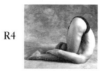

R5

R6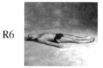

Postures

THE BALANCING PRACTICE

This practice may be used when all the others have been learned. To complete this within 15 minutes will mean that either all the postures are easy fro you, or you are rushing. Best to save this practice for a day when you have a little more time, and until you have learned all the postures.

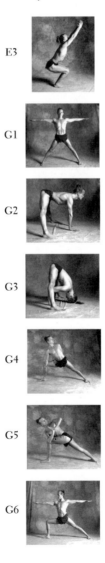

E3

G1

G2

G3

G4

G5

G6

O1

O2

O3

O4

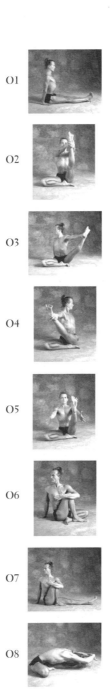

O5

O6

O7

O8

Postures

O9

O12

O13

R1

R2

R3

R4

R5

R6

15-Minute Yoga

MEDITATION

Meditation is the very heart of yoga practice. The practice of meditation begins with the practice of the postures. They bring stability to the body, harmony to the nerves, and quietness to the mind. They are the beginning of the practice of meditation. For meditation to bear its richest fruit it requires absolute stillness of body, and absolute continuity of attention. Most yoga postures cannot be held long enough. Those that can be held do not guarantee the required stability or continuity of attention. Therefore extended meditation is best practiced in a sitting posture.

There are two basic approaches to meditation. One, based on one-pointedness, requires a supporting context only available away from the world—in an ashram or a monastery. The other, based on awareness, requires no special situation. The basis of each, however, is the same. Both depend upon developing the ability to direct attention to subtle, internal stimuli. Both depend on concentration. In the first approach this is developed to an extreme degree, where all other stimuli are systematically rejected. In the second approach concentration is utilized as a basis for inquiring into the activity arising and passing within the chosen context of awareness. It is this approach that is accessible to those leading a normal, daily life.

The notion that meditation is a state in which there are no thoughts is both true and misleading. A state in which no thoughts actually arise is the result of advanced concentrative meditation. Advanced awareness or insight meditation sometimes gives the impression of thoughtlessness, but this is a trick of perception. Thoughts are still arising, but they do not trigger associative thoughts, and the spaces between them seem so vast as to imply that the mind has stopped generating thoughts. The spaces seem vast because the usual referents that constantly pass through the mind, giving a sense of continual change or time passing, are no longer there. Trying to impose stillness on the mind is hopeless. The mind slows down and comes to rest in its own time.

This process is begun in the postures—the dynamic, active aspect of yoga. It is brought to fruition in the stillness of a sitting posture—the still, passive aspect of the practice. This is where the effect of the dynamic aspect is assimilated and becomes a valuable seed of transformation. Without stillness at the end yoga is not only incomplete, but can bring about distur-bance and imbalance. The physical and psychic blocks that have been released by the posture work must be resolved in the quiet and safe solitude of our practice. If this is not allowed to happen the blocks can remain unre-solved and create instability in our lives.

Resolution requires a very definite quality of awareness. It must be stable, tranquil, open, direct, full, and immediate. Stability means that the mind is no longer prone to react to the slightest stimulus. Tranquillity means that the mind is no longer in a grasping, greedy mode. Openness means that it is not looking for anything in particular. Directness means that the mind is no longer using its considerable techniques for distancing itself from the actu-ality of that which is. Fullness means that it is fully engaged in its activity. Finally, immediateness means that there is no hesitation, no prevarication, no evasiveness in engaging the subject. These qualities are initiated through judicious practice of the postures. They must, however, be refined in stillness.

To promote this quality of awareness we use the natural activity of the breath to harness the natural activity of the mind. The breath is the most fundamental expression of our life—and without which we soon have none. It is also a natural and accurate expression of the essential quality of reality. It is a single, dynamic continuum with two apparently opposite aspects that complement, create, and define each other. This is the essence of the core dynamic of reality. To pay attention to, and become absorbed by the breath is both to access the most fundamental arena of our life, and to resonate with the deepest pulse of all that is.

When we use our breath as the seed with which to focus our attention, concentrate our minds and clarify our awareness we remain in touch with that which is. We also do not impose anything on that which is. We simply acknowledge, embrace, and accept it. In doing so we no longer impose our projections, our intentions, our ambitions onto that which is. Thus we become more fully and deeply a part of that which is: a passing wave in the tide of its dynamic fluidity. The breath is a perfect tool for learning the meaning and importance of surrender.

During the practice of the postures our attention has become used to following the breath. Now, without the need to consider the challenging subtleties of muscular adjustment and integrity, it can become clarified by it. Following the breath is a simple but potent practice. But if it is not approached judiciously it can be almost impossible. The rhythmic flow of the breath is so consistent, so subtle in its variety that the habituated, everyday mind is not capable of staying with it for more than a few seconds. It is too addicted to intense, exciting, constantly changing stimuli. So the conditioned, analyzing, grasping mind must be replaced by an unconditioned, accepting, unclinging mind. This takes time to establish, even after the powerful effect of the posture practice. So the sitting practice of cultivating meditative awareness must be approached, like the postures, step-by-step.

The steps required to stabilize, focus, refine, and clarify the mind are like bricks in a wall rather than stones on a pavement. To reach the next we do not leave the previous behind. Each one rests upon the sure and steady support of those beneath it. So we take our time to establish each step, to secure ourselves in it. Then, and only then from that stability, do we move on to the next step. Again the next step is not something separate from the one before, but one that takes it into itself. Each step is a subset of those that come after it. So, when the last step is established, the first is not only there, but more fully so. This is the utilization of the step-by-step progression that is the core of the classical practice of yoga.

The mind is very rich. But its treasures are not all obvious. In fact its most valuable treasures are rarely glimpsed. To find them it is not a question of throwing away its lesser gems but of allowing them to resolve themselves. The dynamism, speed, creativity, and imagination of the mind are phenomenal. Harnessed by the will they are incredibly productive. When they overpower the will they can be equally destructive. In yoga we are not really concerned with these qualities of the mind. We are opening to its hidden gems—its stillness, its openness, its clarity. But we cannot impose them. We cannot force them to be present. They come, quite naturally, when we give up our habituated need to move the mind, to express its dynamism, and to create with it. This giving up is not so easy. It takes practice for the mind to be satisfied by the subtlety of its deeper, richer layers.

It is important, then, not to be unrealistic and expect too much. Sitting still and observing the breath usually reveals one thing more clearly and consistently than anything else: that the mind cannot resist moving, and it seems to care little where or how it moves. Becoming aware of the incessant movement of the mind is the first step in going beyond it. It is not a sign of incompetence. We have to learn to be able to bear the mind's vagaries before we are able to access its inner secrets. By paying attention to the flow of the breath we harness that tendency of the mind to move to something that is moving continuously too, but in a very consistent, rhythmic, and stable manner. This consistency, rhythm and stability then affect the mind. It becomes more stable, rhythmic, and consistent. This takes time—and practice.

After the instructions for how to sit to meditate (overleaf), eight steps for establishing the mind in its innate stillness and clarity by using awareness of your breath are outlined. Do not hurry from one step to the next. Give each one enough time to establish itself. This might be anywhere from 5 to 15 minutes for any or each of the steps. In the beginning you may not be able to get past the first few steps. Be honest with yourself. If you skip from one step to the next without having established it well, you will simply be playing out the speed and grasping of the mind. You will just be going through the motions of the practice. Instead give your mind the time it needs to establish itself in stillness step by step. This not only means following the step-by-step sequence in your practice session. It also means allowing your mind to develop its capacity for concentration, internalization, and silence over time. It may take many months of daily practice before it is even worth attempting the sixth and seventh steps. When you have reached your current capacity in any practice session, release the mind by reversing the steps until you are back where you started: finishing *always* in the eighth step.

177

Adepts Pose

This posture stabilizes the body, quietens the nerves, and stills the mind. Most people will benefit from sitting to the front of a cushion, pile of blankets or something else that will give you the height to have a stable base with both shins supported at the knees.

If it is comfortable you may sit in the full lotus position, *but* take *great* care in entering and leaving the position to avoid straining your knees.

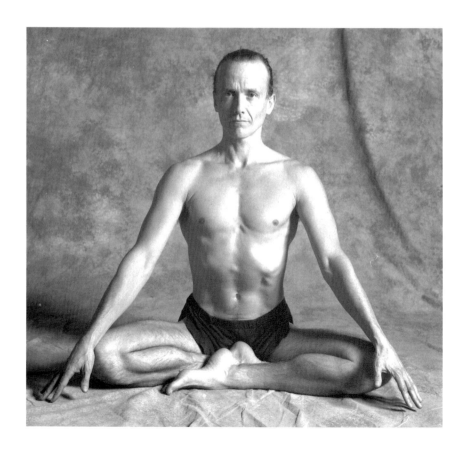

1. Sit on the floor with your legs in front of you.
2. Bend one leg and, keeping the knee soft, place the heel against the center of your pubic bone, or, if comfortable, deeper under against the perineum.
3. Bend the other leg and put the heel just in front of your other one.
4. Relax your legs, pelvis, and abdomen.
5. Come to the front edge of your buttock bones, and stabilize your base with both shins well supported on the floor, or on some raised support.
6. Gently lift your ribcage away from your pelvis, lengthening your spine.
7. Keeping your armpits up, roll your shoulders back and drop your shoulderblades down your back.
8. Look straight ahead with your attention within.

Hold your body still and follow the flow of your breathing with the core of your body soft.

MEDITATION: THE CENTERING PRACTICE

Step 1: Establishing the base

Pay attention to the quality of your base. Feel the stability provided by the triangular base of your buttock bones and shins and their contact with the floor or cushion. Let go of any tension that you find in your legs and pelvis. Allow your mind to be absorbed by the sensations in your lower body, so that it absorbs their stability and stillness.

Step 2: Relaxing the body

From your awareness of your base in your pelvis, allow this awareness to extend itself up the spine to the top of your head; relax your whole body without collapsing into a slumping posture. Allow your mind to be fully absorbed by the sensations of your body relaxing, with a feeling of the muscles melting downwards into and out of the stability of your pelvis.

Step 3: Contacting the spine from the base

While feeling the complementary dynamic of your outer body relaxing down into the stability of your pelvis, become aware of the natural tendency of the spine to elongate itself upward, feeling it rise effortlessly upward out of the pelvis. Allow your mind to be fully absorbed by the floating sensation of the spine as it rises in response to your body letting go more and more fully within the dynamic stability of your posture.

Step 4: Releasing the core

Within your awareness of the inner, complementary dynamic of your posture rising from the stability of your base, allow your attention to release the pelvic floor of any tension, especially in the anus. At the same time allow the brain to soften more and more deeply, so that your eyes and ears are melting into your brain and the softening in the brain and pelvis meet each other, as your core opens more and more fully within the dynamic stability of your posture.

Step 5: Tuning into the breath

As you sit within the stable dynamic of your posture rooted in your pelvis, and while you are aware of the open quality of your core, feel the flow of your breath as it comes and goes. Do not be concerned with how your breath is flowing; simply be aware of it, allowing your mind to be fully absorbed by the spontaneous rhythm of your breathing within the dynamic stability of your posture.

Step 6: Releasing the exhalation

Within the stable, open dynamic of your sitting give especial attention to the exhalation, allowing it to completely expel itself without being imposed on by the following inhalation. Make sure that each exhalation has finished before beginning the inhalation. This does not mean that you should force the lungs to empty, or deliberately prolong the exhalation—simply make sure that the exhalation is not being restricted in any way.

Step 7: Supporting the flow of the breath

Within the stable, open dynamic of your sitting feel the impact that releasing your exhalation has. Feel the increasing stability and fluidity of your inhalation and exhalation, without any imposition. Simply allow your mind to be absorbed by the sensations that arise from the flow of your breathing within the dynamic stability of your posture.

Step 8: Sitting quietly with yourself

Simply sit quietly with yourself, enjoying the play of sensation that your body and your environment bring.

CHOOSING A YOGA TEACHER

The world is full of yoga teachers. Some trained, others not. Some superficially trained, some untrained but with a deep and practical understanding based on experience. Some who teach for love of yoga. Some who teach for love of human beings. Some who teach for love of themselves. Some who teach one style, some another. It can be hard to know where to go and who to try. The most important thing is whether you are able to trust the person teaching you, and whether communication actually occurs. Some teachers can be full of knowledge, charisma or both, and though they can overawe us they cannot reach us in a way that leaves us with anything of value. It is a matter of trial and error. There is no formula that can lead you to a teacher, but some things can help.

Iyengar Yoga teachers have been well trained in the structural precision of the method of yoga, and focus mostly on correct and safe technique. They are useful guides in ensuring that you are doing the postures correctly.

Vinniyoga teachers put greater emphasis on finding a practice that exactly suits the student, and focusing more on sensitivity and breathing. They are useful guides in ensuring that you are being sensitive to yourself in your practice.

Ashtanga Vinyasa Yoga teachers tend to be dedicated practitioners with a more intuitive understanding that can be very inspiring. The focus is more on experience and doing than on understanding or knowledge. They are useful guides in ensuring that you go deep into your practice and develop the continuity and stamina that deep internalization requires.

There are, of course, many other teaching styles and individual teachers who have something to offer. In selecting a teacher or teaching style it is not a matter of right and wrong. No teacher knows everything. No teacher knows nothing. No teacher can communicate what they know to everybody and no teacher can reach no-one. If we are open, sensitive, and take responsibility for what we do without surrendering our judgment (while surrendering our assumptions at the same time), we can benefit from any yoga teacher. It is best to try a few before committing to one teacher or one style. To change teachers continuously can lead to confusion as they will all say something different. Even when they are saying the same thing but in different ways, the student is not always able to tell this.

A very beneficial combination is to occasionally go to a good Iyengar teacher to refine your technique, while occasionally going to an Ashtanga Vinyasa teacher for encouragement, support, and the power of a group dynamic. However yoga is a personal practice. Going to class is always a compromise—though one that is definitely necessary occasionally. In a class we cannot go at our own pace, nor can we follow our intuitive sense of what is right in that particular moment. But, and more so in the beginning, we can learn or experience things we would not in our own practice, where we can then apply them.

The relationship between yoga student and teacher is unique. It is one in which both the teacher and student come to a deeper awareness of the student. This can create a closeness and intimacy that has not had the usual growth pattern of shared experience and knowledge. It is an intimacy based more on a deep, intuitive familiarity rather than a conscious knowing. This can be a little awkward to deal with. It is important for a student to remember that even though the teacher can and does touch you very deeply, they do not actually know anything about you that you have not communicated. They may sense from your expression or your body language that you are sad, but they do not know what you are sad about, nor why it makes you sad. It is important not to project on to teachers what is not there. They are not all-seeing and all-knowing. They are fallible human beings whose technical expertise does not necessarily go hand-in-hand with a deep understanding of the human condition, nor empathy with individual human beings.

In the beginning it is necessary to go to classes, but as time passes and your practice matures this should happen less and less. The technique of the method is in fact quite simple. There will be moments when some principle will become clear to you, and you will then be able to apply it in any posture at any time. Eventually your practice will clarify for you, even if only on an unconscious level, all of the principles underlying the method. Then not only are you ready and able to continue your journey alone, but it will feel less and less appropriate to go to a class and be told by someone else what to do. However, as you go deeper into your practice feedback becomes more important than instruction. It is easy to take a wrong track that can lead to unwanted places. Yoga is a powerful practice that amplifies whatever we bring to it. If it is working for us life itself will give us that feedback by becoming more and more harmonious, more and more rewarding. On the other hand life can also tell us that we are misusing the practice by making us feel more and more self important, immune to feedback, and narrow-minded in our approach to ourselves and to life. We all need to allow the "guru function" into our lives if we are to go deeply into yoga. This means being open to the feedback life gives us, and to be constantly thinking about and questioning our conclusions, motivations, understanding, and assumptions.

It can help immensely to have a friend who has already gone further down the path, and to whom we are open on this level. The quality of feedback that we require does not have to come from a guru, or wise teacher. Life itself can provide it for us if we approach our practice with a genuine honesty and open sensitivity. Then everything that we do becomes a reflection of our inner state in the mirror of life: not only what we do, but what happens to us also. Our every action, thought, feeling, and circumstance can reveal the quality of our attitudes, assumptions, and motivation if we look upon life as a mirror—and if we are truly willing to see what is revealed there, no matter how much it does or does not fit in with our desires, hopes, and expectations.

Besides a wise and seasoned friend, the best sources of outside feedback are the people to whom you are closest in life: lovers, children, parents. It is in our relationships to others, rather than in our physical prowess, that the effects and benefits of our practice are revealed. Are we becoming closer, more intimate, more sensitive and responsive to those we love, or are we becoming more isolated, alienated, and aloof?

ABOUT THE AUTHOR

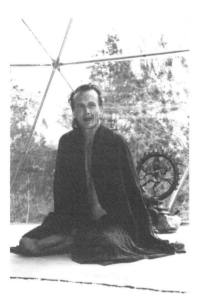

Godfrey began his yoga practice in 1973 at the age of 16. He has practiced almost daily since then, and has made yoga the foundation of his life. He has studied with many teachers, from both the East and West: most notably B.K.S. Iyengar of Pune, and B.N.S. Iyengar of Mysore. His participation in the Zen Buddhist "Kanzeon Sangha" as a student of Soten Genpo Roshi has been the biggest influence on his understanding of the subtlety and implications of yoga as a spiritual practice. He has been teaching yoga since 1979 and teaching yoga exclusively since 1989.

He is the author of a general introduction to yoga: *The Elements of Yoga* and a practical beginners' guide: *Hatha Yoga Breath by Breath*. He is also the author of *Dynamic Yoga*, outlining his personal approach to the practice, which blends the precision of Iyengar Yoga, the dynamism of Ashtanga Vinyasa Yoga, and the sensitivity of Vinniyoga into a single whole. It reveals and makes immediately accessible the power of yoga and its inherent simplicity. He has also made many audio and video tapes, and has self-published a number of small booklets on specific aspects of yoga. Having been Director of Yoga at The Life Centre in London, he now runs a dedicated Yoga Training Centre in Ibiza, offering courses year round for all levels—beginners to trainee teachers.

If you would like to be included on Godfrey's mailing list please write to:

Windfire Yoga
36 Stanbridge Road
London SW15 1DX
or telephone 08700 780 239

For detailed current information about Godfrey's workshops, retreats, and teacher training courses, visit his website at:

www.windfireyoga.com

5612